Neuropsychological Interventions for Children - Volume 1

Caroline de Oliveira Cardoso
Natália Martins Dias
Editors

Neuropsychological Interventions for Children - Volume 1

From Early-Preventive Stimulation to Rehabilitation

Springer

Editors
Caroline de Oliveira Cardoso
Universidade Feevale
Novo Hamburgo, Rio Grande do Sul, Brazil

Natália Martins Dias
Universidade Federal de Santa Catarina
Florianópolis, Santa Catarina, Brazil

ISBN 978-3-031-53585-7 ISBN 978-3-031-53586-4 (eBook)
https://doi.org/10.1007/978-3-031-53586-4

The translation was done with the help of an artificial intelligence machine translation tool. A subsequent human revision was done primarily in terms of content.

Translation from the Portuguese language edition: "Intervenção Neuropsicológica Infantil: Da Estimulação Precoce-Preventiva à Reabilitação" by Caroline de Oliveira Cardoso and Natália Martins Dias, © Natália Dias and Caroline de Oliveira Cardoso 2019. Published by Pearson. All Rights Reserved.

This Springer imprint is published by the registered company Springer Nature Switzerland AG
The registered company address is: Gewerbestrasse 11, 6330 Cham, Switzerland

Paper in this product is recyclable.

Foreword to the Brazilian Edition

Development is a continuous process that is influenced by brain maturation, which is a complex phenomenon involving genetic, structural, and neuroplasticity aspects, and environmental and social factors (family interaction styles, culture, socioeconomic level, and literacy methods) that play a crucial role in cognition. The professional working in the field of Developmental Neuropsychology analyzes the domain he or she is working in from three main components, all complex: the dynamic developmental process of the organism, the potential threats to development that the organism is subject to (including the impact of diseases/disorders and of experiences in adverse environments), and the available assessment and intervention strategies. In this sense, training for education, health, and social care professionals needs to be reviewed, as highlighted by the National Early Childhood Plan (Brazil), in order to broaden and deepen the knowledge base of these professionals, enhancing the qualities and skills to develop their practice. In this scenario, Developmental Neuropsychology should be considered as an essential part and not just a background.

The relevance of this book to address the contributions of research to the practice of the professional who deals with the specificities of childhood has immense value because the book addresses in an interdisciplinary way aspects of assessment and intervention in different contexts, i.e., research, clinical, and school contexts. The selection of chapters brings a unique characteristic in works currently available, written by professionals who make the intersection between areas of knowledge.

Part 1 – Theoretical and Practical Foundation on Child Neuropsychological Assessment and Intervention – presents us with six chapters that address the premises of neuropsychological assessment; of intervention in childhood, with an important differentiation of the terminologies applied to this area and its methods; of stimulation in the school context and the relevance of activities such as music, dance, singing, and physical activities, among others; and the issues of the relevance of reporting and returning results, which has been the target of many doubts and questions from professionals in their practice. There is constant pointing by the authors of the information provided by parents and teachers about the impact of the condition on the child's daily life, of the importance of considering observation protocols as a tool for understanding the presence, nature, and extent of the child's life commitments, as well as understanding the potential of the direct and indirect effect of a given condition on that child with whom the professional is dealing. This is an important point that developmental neuropsychologists have been pushing for decades. I often use a phrase in my classes to illustrate this: "More than saying whether the child has (for example) dyslexia is saying *who* that child with dyslexia is". And that has been a very salient point throughout this book.

In Part 2 – Stimulation and Rehabilitation – there are seven chapters that address neuropsychological intervention of specific functions such as attention, memory, executive functions, social and emotional skills, mathematical skills, and reading comprehension, with lots of information for health professionals and tips for parents and teachers. This part also highlights the importance of early stimulation, one of the most discussed factors today, especially considering the high prevalence in some countries of children with learning disabilities and behavior problems. The importance of early intervention to increase children's opportunities, especially those lacking environmental experiences, has been constantly highlighted by the authors of this book, through their research, so that the government may consider this in the implementation of policies for Early Childhood Education in Brazil and other countries. According to authors from around the world, models of intervention and stimulation require professionals from all disciplines to work together to bring out the many areas of knowledge needed to support children with difficulties or impairments in the course of development.

Therefore, this work brings this immense contribution, because, in addition to what was exposed above, it reaffirms what is recommended by the National Plan for Early Childhood (PNPI; Brazil), which attributes research a strategic role in reaching its objectives, in the continuity and expansion of its goals, in the extension to new sectors or areas that, in the coming years, will demand attention and in the improvement of the quality of attention to the child. The accessible language of the chapters' is another differential, as it allows professionals from other areas, such as education, to consult chapters of interest.

I congratulate the book's organizers, Caroline de Oliveira Cardoso and Natalia Martins Dias, young researchers who have already contributed to the advancement of Developmental Neuropsychology in our country. The book fills a gap in the area by meeting the demand for training and information with robust scientific evidence.

Department of Psychology
Universidade Federal da Bahia
Salvador, Bahia, Brazil

Monica Carolina Miranda

Acknowledgments

"*A whole book about intervention*!" This was our goal when the idea of setting up this partnership came up. A partnership that combined the scientific interest of two young researchers with experience in developing interventions, authors of PIAFEx and PENcE, and the concern in making available material with practical tips, truly useful.

From this initial idea came not just one, but two works of "Neuropsychological Interventions for Children":

- Volume 1: "From early-preventive stimulation to rehabilitation"
- Volume 2: "Applications and Interfaces"

From our experience in the development, application, and evaluation of intervention programs in childhood, we believe that we have assembled in these two books a unique team, which will certainly make this book a reference in the area of child neuropsychology. We thank the fellow authors, experts in their respective areas, who readily agreed to collaborate with us, writing chapters rich in research data, professional experience, and rationale for practice for both books.

We thank, above all, the organizers of the "Neuropsychology in Clinical Practice Collection", where this work was initially and originally published, in Brazil, and Springer, which gave us international visibility. This partnership certainly brings a great contribution to the development of neuropsychology in Brazil and worldwide.

Caroline de Oliveira Cardoso
Natália Martins Dias
Volume Editors

Contents

Contributors

Mariana Abuhamad Psychologist from the Universidade Federal do Paraná (UFPR), master in psychology in the line Neuropsychological evaluation and rehabilitation by UFPR. Specialist in Neuropsychology by the Federal Council of Psychology (CFP). Owner of the company Cognos – Cognitive Stimulation Materials.

Nara Côrtes Andrade Professor at the Department of Psychology of the Universidade Federal de Juiz de Fora, Brazil. She is also an associate researcher at Harvard University. PhD in Experimental Psychology from Universidade de São Paulo (USP), completed a master's in Developmental Neuropsychology at the Universidade Federal da Bahia and a postdoctoral research program at Harvard University. She has been serving in leadership positions in professional organizations in neuropsychology, such as the International Neuropsychological Society (INS), Latin American Neuropsychological Society (SLAN, Brazil representative) and Neuropsychology Committee of the National Association of Research and Graduate Studies in Psychology (ANPEPP), Brazil. She is currently Consulting editor of the Neuropsychology Journal (APA) and Revista Neuropsicología Latinoamericana (SLAN).

Marco Antônio Arruda Child and adolescent neurologist, PhD, Visiting Professor of Universidade Estadual de Campinas, and Director of Glia Institute.

Helena Vellinho Corso Psychopedagogue. Master in Educational Psychology from the Postgraduate Program of the Faculty of Education of the Universidade Federal do Rio Grande do Sul (UFRGS, Brazil) and PhD in Psychology from the Postgraduate Program of the Institute of Psychology, UFRGS. Professor at the Faculty of Education of UFRGS. Researcher and professor of the Postgraduate Program of the School of Education, UFRGS.

Luciana Vellinho Corso Psychopedagogue, Licensed in Pedagogy, Universidade Federal do Rio Grande do Sul (UFRG, Brazil). Master in Education, Flinders University, Australia. PhD in Education, UFRGS. Associate Professor of the Postgraduate Program of the School of Education, UFRGS. Researcher and member of the Psychopedagogical Board of the Attention Deficit/Hyperactivity Disorder Program (PRODAH), Clinical Hospital (HCPOA), RS, Brazil.

Narahyana Bom de Araújo Psychologist. Master and PhD in Mental Health from the Universidade Federal do Rio de Janeiro (UFRJ). Specialist in Neuropsychology by the Santa Casa de Misericórdia of Rio de Janeiro (RJ). Psychologist at the Policlínica Naval Nossa Senhora da Glória- PNNSG/MB.

Ariane Cristina Ramello de Carvalho Psychologist from the Pontifícia Universidade Católica de Goiás (PUC-GO). Master and PhD in Developmental Disorders at Universidade Presbiteriana Mackenzie (UPM). Specialist in Neuropsychology by PUC-GO. Professor in the postgraduate course in Neuropsychology at Universidade São Francisco. Clinical Neuropsychologist.

Chrissie Ferreira de Carvalho Professor at the Psychology Department of the Universidade Federal de Santa Catarina (UFSC, Brazil). She has a master degree and a PhD in Developmental Psychology by the Universidade Federal da Bahia and completed postdoctoral studies at the Laboratory for Developmental Studies at Harvard University. Currently is coordinator of the Cognitive and School Neuropsychology Laboratory (LANCE).

Jerusa Fumagalli de Salles Speech Therapist and a Full Professor at the Department of Developmental and Personality Psychology, Institute of Psychology, at Universidade Federal do Rio Grande do Sul (UFRGS, Brazil). She has a M.S. degree and a PhD in Psychology at the same university. She is also a Professor in the Graduate Program in Psychology at UFRGS. She has a Research Productivity Scholarship granted by CNPq (Brazilian research governmental organization) and coordinates the Center for Studies in Cognitive Neuropsychology (Neurocog). She is the head of the Department of Developmental and Personality Psychology and also an associate member of the Technical-Scientific Council of the National Science for Education Network (CpE).

Flavia dos Passos Fonseca Graduated in Psychology from the Pontifícia Universidade Católica do Rio Grande do Sul (PUCRS). Post-graduate specialization in Cognitive Behavioral Therapy (PUCRS).

Rochele Paz Fonseca Psychologist and Speech Therapist. Specialist in Neuropsychology. Master in Developmental Psychology (UFRGS). PhD in Psychology (Neuropsychology), UFRGS / Université de Montréal. Post-Doctorate in Neurosciences and Clinical Psychology (PUC-Rio), Neuroradiology (UFRJ) and Biomedical Sciences (Université de Montréal). Full Professor at Medicine

Department, Universidade Federal de Minas Gerais – Post-Graduate Program of Child and Adolescent Health. Coordinator of the Clinical and Experimental Neuropsychology Group (GNCE). Coordination member of the Technical-Scientific Council of the Science for Education Network (CpE) and the Brazilian Neuropsychology Network. Productivity researcher 1C of CNPq. President of the Brazilian Society of Neuropsychology (SBNp 2019–2023). Member-at-large of the Board of Governors of the International Neuropsychological Society (INS). Founding partner at Conectare NeuroPsi – Service, training and connections in Neuropsychology.

Hosana Alves Gonçalves Psychologist from the Pontifícia Universidade Católica do Rio Grande do Sul (PUCRS). Master and PhD Psychology from PUCRS with a doctoral internship at the University of Salamanca (Spain). Works as a clinical neuropsychologist in private practice and is a founding partner at Conectare NeuroPsi-Service, training and connections in Neuropsychology.

Tatiana Pontrelli Mecca Psychologist from the Universidade Presbiteriana Mackenzie (UPM). Master, PhD, with post-doctorate, in Developmental Disorders from UPM. She works as a professor at Mental Health Departament in Faculty of Medical Sciences, Santa Casa de São Paulo, Brazil.

Janice da Rosa Pureza Psychologist. Master and PhD in Psychology – Postgraduate Program in Psychology from the Pontifícia Universidade Católica do Rio Grande do Sul (PUCRS) – Concentration Area Human Cognition. Specialization in Neuropsychology from the Universidade Luterana do Brazil (ULBRA). Training in Early Intervention – children from 0 to 3 years – Phoniatrics Clinic / Santo Antônio Children's Hospital (Porto Alegre/RS). Collaborator of the Clinical and Experimental Neuropsychology Group (GNCE) – PUCRS. Works in the areas of child neurodevelopment and neuropsychology of learning. Works with clinical psychology and child neuropsychology and is a founding partner at Conectare NeuroPsi – Service, training and connections in Neuropsychology.

Bruna Evaristo Scheffer Psychologist. Master in Psychology (Human Cognition) from the Pontifícia Universidade Católica do Rio Grande do Sul (PUCRS, Brazil). Psychotherapist in private clinic.

Alessandra Gotuzo Seabra Psychologist from the Universidade de São Paulo (USP, Brazil), Master, PhD, with post-doctorate, in Experimental Psychology from the USP. She works in the postgraduate program in Human Development Sciences at Universidade Presbiteriana Mackenzie, Brazil. CNPq research productivity scholar. Coordinator of the Child Neuropsychology Group and psychologist at the Institute of Neuropsychology and Human Development – INDH.

Nicolle Zimmermann Psychologist. Master in Psychology – Human Cognition by the Pontifícia Universidade Católica do Rio Grande do Sul (PUCRS). Doctor in Sciences (Neuroradiology) by the Universidade Federal do Rio de Janeiro. Specialist in Principles and Practices in Clinical Research by Harvard University. Schema Therapist by Wainer Psicologia/International Society for Schema Therapy.

About the Editors

Caroline de Oliveira Cardoso Psychologist, graduated from Pontifícia Universidade Católica do Rio Grande do Sul (PUCRS), specialist in Neuropsychology (Projecto), Master and PhD in Psychology, emphasis on Human Cognition (PUCRS). Professor of the Psychology Course at Universidade Feevale, Brazil. Permanent teacher of the Academic Master's in Psychology at Universidade Feevale. Coordinator of the Research and Intervention Laboratory in School and Developmental Neuropsychology. Member of the board of the Brazilian Society of Neuropsychology – SBNp (2019–2025) and member of the "Neuropsychology" Working Group of the National Association of Researchers in Psychology (ANPEPP). She works as a psychologist and clinical neuropsychologist and is a founding partner of Conectare NeuroPsi – Service, training and connections in Neuropsychology.

Natália Martins Dias Psychologist, graduated from Universidade São Franscisco. Master and PhD, with post-doctorate, in Developmental Disorders from Universidade Presbiteriana Mackenzie, São Paulo, Brazil. Professor of the Department of Psychology at the Universidade Federal de Santa Catarina – UFSC, Brazil. Coordinator of the Cognitive and School Neuropsychology Laboratory – LANCE. Member of the board of the Brazilian Society of Neuropsychology – SBNp (2019–2025). Associated researcher of the National Science for Education Network – CpE. CNPq Research Productivity Scholar.

Part I
Theoretical and Practical Foundation on Child Neuropsychological Assessment and Intervention

Chapter 1
Neuropsychological Assessment and Its Role in Directing the Intervention

Natália Martins Dias and Alessandra Gotuzo Seabra

As an interdisciplinary science, neuropsychology has a broad scope of action, with various areas of practice and research that require conceptual perspectives, theoretical models, assessment tools, and specific interventions. Within this scope, child neuropsychology is characterized by specifically addressing the understanding of the relationship between neurological and psychological functioning, with the study of neuropsychological functions from the beginning of the life cycle to adolescence. It is therefore essential to understand child development and the influences of genetic, medical, environmental, behavioral, and sociocultural aspects on this development (Baron, 2004).

Historically, interest in understanding the cognitive sequelae of neurological injuries in children only began in the 1960s. At the same time, the need to understand typical development has also strengthened, and currently, the field of child neuropsychology has compiled a large scope of knowledge (Baron, 2004). Advances have been observed in understanding typical neurological development (e.g., Malloy-Diniz et al., 2017), sequelae of neurological damage (Neri, 2012; Taylor et al., 2010), characteristics of populations with syndromes (Costanzo et al., 2013; Freire & Hazin, 2015) and neurodevelopmental disorders (Narzisi et al., 2013; O'Brien et al., 2010), development of intervention tools (Cardoso et al., 2016; Dias & Seabra, 2013; Thomson et al., 2017), transcultural studies (Uzzell et al., 2013), among others. Similarly, child neuropsychological assessment, the subject of this chapter, has greatly advanced, especially in terms of the development of psychometrically appropriate instruments (e.g., in Brazil, Fonseca et al., 2016; Seabra

N. M. Dias (✉)
Universidade Federal de Santa Catarina, Florianópolis, Santa Catarina, Brazil
e-mail: natalia.m.dias@ufsc.br

A. G. Seabra
Universidade Presbiteriana Mackenzie, São Paulo, Brazil
e-mail: alessandra.seabra@mackenzie.br

C. O. Cardoso, N. M. Dias (eds.), *Neuropsychological Interventions for Children - Volume 1*, https://doi.org/10.1007/978-3-031-53586-4_1

et al., 2013, 2016; Seabra & Dias, 2012a, b). On the other hand, there are still specific areas that lack research and practical tools; for example, ecological tasks, which have greater predictive power in daily life activities, are still almost nonexistent in various contexts of action and countries.

Child neuropsychological assessment has both qualitative and quantitative specificities in relation to adult assessment. It is necessary to deeply understand child development and the expected variability in each area to be assessed. Additionally, it is needed to understand how an injury or neurological dysfunction can impact cognitive functioning at each stage of development, as well as the role of environmental, social, and cultural factors on development. The potential for neurological plasticity, the capacity for reorganization in this still immature system, must be considered, which makes the task quite complex.

Demands for Neuropsychological Assessment in Childhood: Common Complaints and Referral Sources

Some complaints stand out in the referral of children and adolescents for neuropsychological assessment. For example, complaints related to the signs present in various Neurodevelopmental Disorders, such as Autism Spectrum Disorder, Specific Learning Disorder, Attention Deficit/Hyperactivity Disorder, Intellectual Development Disorder, Communication Disorders or Motor Disorders (American Psychiatric Association [APA], 2014), as well as neurological conditions (such as epilepsy, traumatic brain injury), psychiatric and behavioral complaints. Thus, neuropsychological assessment in childhood and adolescence is of great help in diagnosing these conditions.

One of the main sources of referrals is the ***school*** in the case of children/adolescents with learning or behavior difficulties. The referred individuals may have already seen other professionals or have been primarily referred to the neuropsychologist. School complaints may be related to neuropsychological problems or not (as occurs in learning difficulties). Either way, the neuropsychological assessment can help clarify the complaint and guide the necessary referrals. The most common reports are of problems with academic learning and/or behavior problems, especially when externalizing.

The ***family*** is another important source of referral. It is possible that the child or adolescent manifests, in the family context, difficulties and behaviors not observed in other places, such as school. The differences in reports between parents and teachers, already well documented in the literature (Major & Seabra-Santos, 2013, 2014; Martoni et al., 2016), should not be seen as imprecision on the part of the informants, as they may be due to the differences that exist in each context, such as the various cognitive demands and the specific social situations to which individuals are exposed.

Another point is that the neuropsychological assessment can have different focuses depending on the examinee's age. The assessment usually focuses on language, cognitive and motor developments, and basic socio-emotional skills in preschoolers. In school-age children, the focus tends to be on skills related to the school environment and its demands, including the first skills related to reading, writing and math, attention and executive functions, emotional control and social functioning. Adolescents are also assessed for academic progress, emotional and behavioral control, and social functioning (Hale & Fiorello, 2004; Semrud-Clikeman & Ellison, 2009).

Planning the Assessment and the Tools of the Process: How to Collect Information?

Even before selecting strategies and instruments for the assessment process, it is essential to have clarity of its objectives. In the clinical field, one can mention (based on Miotto, 2016):

1. Assistance in nosological diagnosis.
2. Greater understanding of the nature and extent of the impairments (cognitive, emotional and behavioral) presented by the individual.
3. Mapping of the individual's cognitive functioning through the outlining of their neuropsychological profile ("peaks and valleys" profile).
4. Foundation and proposition of interventions aimed at the specific needs and impairments of the patient.
5. Monitoring and measuring the effects of the intervention (or others, such as medication, surgical procedure or from other professionals), being able to feed back into the process and suggest new directions for the intervention.

In other words, beyond hypothesis testing and profile raising, neuropsychological assessment is the first step (and a fundamental step) in intervention planning. In this sense, the neuropsychologist needs to ensure that their strategies and tools will provide useful, quantity and quality information to guide the entire process.

Indeed, child neuropsychological assessment should not be defined as a simple process of applying instruments or, from an even more restrictive perspective, of a single instrument. Currently, far beyond seeking correlations between scores on a test and neurological functioning, neuropsychological assessment should allow drawing a profile of the examinee, in which the results in tests do play a critical role but are interpreted in the light of a global context, which includes clinical observations, the individual's history, their sociocultural context and information from other sources. The joint analysis of all these aspects will provide child neuropsychological assessment with utility as a guide for decision-making and school, clinical or family interventions (Baron, 2004).

The whole process begins with the ***Clinical Interview or Anamnesis***, a common practice in the field that aims to mainly understand and deepen the demand, as well as clarify the clinical history and all set of cognitive, emotional and behavioral complaints and their impact on the patient's life, besides, of course, gathering information about the development and functioning of the patient. A model of clinical interview is provided in Annex I of this chapter. In child care, this stage is carried out with the guardians. In the case of teenagers, the initial interview to obtain information about the patient's development history and the complaint is also carried out with the guardians. However, a second interview session may be conducted with the teenager in an attempt to also encompass their perspective on their difficulties, how they experience them and how they impact their life and complement information from the interview with the guardians.

After the clinical interview, which generally takes place in one to two sessions, the neuropsychologist already has material that allows them to raise hypotheses. Testing them is the second step of the process, with the application of instruments for skills assessment, which we will designate here as the ***hypothesis testing stage***. The selection of assessment instruments should be careful, not only due to the smaller number of options available in some countries for this age range but also because, in children, there is a tendency for less precision and validity of the measures (Baron, 2004; Seabra et al., 2012). This makes it essential for the examiner to observe the characteristics of the child, unite different sources of information and offer the child situations in which the target behaviors can be observed (clinical tasks). In this process, the set of techniques and tools that can help the neuropsychologist obtain information is described in the topics below. The first of these tools refers to the neuropsychological tests or tasks.

Neuropsychological Tests or Tasks

They allow quantifying the child's performance and interpreting it in relation to a normative standard (such as age or schooling, for example). It is an objective form of assessment that uses standardized materials and procedures.

The use of standardized instruments is important, and the professional should pay attention to its psychometric qualities, the norms provided, and the normative sample, as well as to the studies of validity evidence that should provide information about which constructs the test evaluates and what the relationships are between such constructs and daily life behaviors of the individual, at home, at school or in other contexts (Baron, 2004).

The results of standardized instruments should be interpreted in a convergent way with each other and with the other information obtained about the child/adolescent. Due to the impurity of the tasks, often a lower performance on a test may not be due to a deficit in the main construct evaluated by the test but rather in other skills necessary for the good performance of the test but secondary in terms of defining the evaluated construct. For example, it is common for a child with a decrease in verbal working memory to have low performance in oral arithmetic subtests, not because she has a real decrease in arithmetic, which is the target construct of the test, but rather due to the problem in verbal working memory. The same child may perform closer to expected if the arithmetic task is visuospatial. It is therefore essential that the neuropsychologist is aware of this pattern of convergence between results to trace the neuropsychological profile of the examinee.

Tracing this profile is one of the main objectives of the use of standardized instruments, as they enable mapping "strengths" and "weaknesses" from structured tasks referenced to a norm (Miotto, 2016). In turn, this functioning profile will be greatly informative to the intervention process.

On one hand, the use of tests or standardized tasks provides objectivity and precision to the evaluation process. On the other hand, one should not dispense with qualitative observations during this psychological assessment process. Thus, the professional should also be aware of the types of errors, self-correction, response patterns, and engagement in the task, among others.

A possible strategy is to start the evaluation with a battery of tests and, after initial results, deepen the evaluation in specific areas. For example, in the Brazilian context, a battery that can be used to evaluate children from 6 to 12 years old is the Brief Child Neuropsychological Assessment Instrument—NEUPSILIN-Inf (Salles et al., 2016). Its application can occur in a single session, from approximately 40 to 60 min. The following areas are evaluated: orientation (temporal and spatial), attention (visual and auditory), perception (visual and of emotions in faces), memory (episodic-semantic visuo-verbal, episodic-semantic verbal, semantic memory and working memory), arithmetic skills, language (oral and written), constructive praxis and executive functions. Another example is the use of the WISC (Rueda et al., 2013) in neuropsychological assessment. The instrument is available in several languages and countries and has been used to outline a cognitive functioning profile from the performance in various subtests. From the results of this first evaluation, the neuropsychologist can plan the continuation of the evaluation based on the observed profile, complementing the process with more specific tasks.

Functional Measures

These measures try to measure behavior in more routine situations as they manifest in daily activities and situations. In general, they are standardized scales or inventories that can be answered by parents, teachers and, in some cases, by the child/adolescent themselves. These tools allow evaluating the occurrence and even quantify behaviors, specific difficulties, and symptoms, among other phenomena targets of the evaluation.

A relevant point to this discussion is that, to be informative to intervention planning, the evaluation process needs to be comprehensive and provide information that complements the neuropsychological functioning profile with an analysis of impact in the "real world" (Miotto, 2016). That is, knowing the individual's behavior and functionality in their daily activities can, even, collaborate in the delimitation of the intervention targets: What are his/her *difficulties in daily life? What are his/her cognitive alterations, and how is this associated with the difficulties or incapacity he/she experiences in school activities or in his/her relationships with peers? What is his/her functional capacity? How does the identified cognitive change impact his/her daily life activities?*

Much of this information can be provided by functional measures. They represent the perception of those who live with the patient (or even the patient himself) about his functioning in the world. It is, in a way, complementary to neuropsychological tasks and tests since it focuses on a different level of analysis; that is, while tests in general focus on the cognitive level, scales and inventories tend to prioritize the behavioral level. The joint analysis provides subsidies to the neuropsychologist for the articulation between different levels of analysis of the individual's functioning.

An interesting aspect regarding functional measures is the generally low agreement between respondents in the case of parents and teachers. Some findings suggest that parents tend to attribute more difficulties or problems to their children when their evaluation is compared to the teacher's. Numerous variables can contribute to this low agreement, such as, for example, different expectations that each evaluator has in relation to the child's behavior, divergent interpretations of the scale items and specific characteristics of the environment in which the observation occurs, which include stimuli, structure, presence of peers and rules. For example, certain behaviors may be more easily observed at school than at home (e.g., is collaborative with other children; can engage attention for a long enough time to finish their tasks among others), making them more accessible to the teacher's evaluation (Major & Seabra-Santos, 2013, 2014; Martoni et al., 2016).

Also, it is worth highlighting the low relationships between functional measures, both answered by parents and by teachers, and performance measures, such as neuropsychological tests and tasks (Martoni et al., 2016; Seabra-Santos & Gaspar, 2012; Toplak et al., 2013). Such findings have often raised questions regarding whether these measures would evaluate the same construct. This low degree of agreement, however, is not necessarily negative. It becomes important to understand the different evaluation situations (more structured in performance tests *versus* functioning in different environments) and try to understand them as complementary. Such situations can even give clues about how the environment can influence or mediate certain behaviors.

Other Information: Parents and Teachers Report

Beyond the information collected by standardized functional measures, other information can be obtained through interviews with parents and teachers. With parents, beyond the anamnesis, which allows the knowledge of the child's developmental history and clinical history, it is still pertinent to gather other information for a better understanding and deepening of the difficulties experienced by the patient. This set of information can be obtained in the initial interview or others during the process. Some information that may be relevant: situations in which the difficulty occurs, the existence of environmental variables that precipitate or aggravate the difficulties or problem behaviors, parents' reaction to such behaviors, among others that investigate family engagement in the process and use of compensatory strategies, such as what the family's involvement in the patient's treatment is, what strategy patient and family use to deal with difficulties and impact of the complaint not only for the patient but for the family (Miotto, 2016).

Regarding information from teachers, they can give valuable tips about aspects associated with the child's learning, their organization for tasks, their engagement and motivation for school learning, as well as their social functioning, such as their relationship with peers and their friendships, disruptive behavior, among others. Observing school tasks and notebooks can also reveal performance patterns that give interesting clues, especially in cases where there are complaints of learning difficulties.

Observation

The basic triad of an evaluation process is completed with observation (tests + interviews + observation). The observation can occur in the clinical context itself, during the performance of activities, for example, to check how the child deals with problems or unexpected events or what kind of strategy they use to solve a given problem (ecological tasks can be very useful here). It allows obtaining information that complements those from tests and interviews.

In addition, standardized observation protocols can still be used to measure the frequency and intensity of behaviors considered relevant in the face of a certain complaint or professional hypothesis. An example is the Assessment Protocol for Children Suspected of Autism Spectrum Disorders (PROTEA-R; Bosa & Salles, 2018), which presents a behavioral assessment protocol in addition to anamnesis interview. The instrument systematizes the clinical evaluation of children suspected of Autism Spectrum Disorder based on the observation and recording of behaviors that are diagnostic criteria of the condition. The evaluation occurs through observation of the child interacting with an adult (parents and/or professional) and using some materials and toys over the course of 3 sessions. The items (behaviors to be observed) are grouped into three dimensions: (1) social interaction, language and communication; (2) relationship with objects and play; and (3) stereotyped and self-injurious behavior.

Furthermore, it is possible to carry out the observation in other environments to check how the child interacts and deals with different situations. In the case of child care, this environment is usually the school, which allows the analysis not only of target behaviors but also of how they interact with the environment.

These sources of information do not exhaust the process and should be weighed against the needs of each case. Other relevant sources are those obtained by other professionals who attend to the child/adolescent, such as speech therapists, neurologists, psychiatrists, and educational psychologists. The integration of all the information obtained should provide the professional with a fairly reasonable understanding of the individual's difficulties.

The process, here described from the minimum stages of ***Clinical Interview/Anamnesis*** and ***Hypothesis Testing*** (including different types of measures), is accompanied and concludes with the application of ***clinical reasoning***, which includes quantitative interpretation, as well as qualitative and articulation between all the findings, seeking to corroborate or refute the hypotheses outlined at the beginning of the process. Here, for example, it is appropriate to revisit the complaint and understand how the functioning profile found from the application of the instruments explains or is associated with the complaint and the difficulties encountered in daily life (functional evaluation), defining therapeutic targets. Once this analysis is done, the neuropsychologist is ready to prepare the report and to provide feedback (see Chap. 6 on these topics). The result of the evaluation should be informative for the intervention process.

Neuropsychological Intervention Based on the Evaluation: The Importance of Outlining the Neuropsychological Profile

Once the neuropsychological profile of the patient is defined, it is possible to understand not only their peculiar pattern of skills and difficulties but also the impact of deficits on their behavior and functionality in daily life. Such a profile to be outlined should map strengths and difficulty points. Considering all these information sources, the neuropsychological profile analysis is not fundamentally based on establishing a diagnosis. Still, it should enable the interpretation of behavior in a comprehensive and multidimensional way. An example of how this profile can be outlined is illustrated in the sequence of this chapter, composing a profile of "peaks" (skills or facilities) and "valleys" (difficulties), which allows a clearer visual inspection both to the neuropsychologist and to his/hers patient and relatives.

The profile can be represented by the neuropsychologist in the form of a graph, to facilitate its visualization. In the assembly of this graph, all scores on tests/tasks are converted into a z-score, a standardized scale where the average is zero and variability is given in terms of standard deviations (SD) around the average. Thus, a score between −1 and 1 (shaded area) corresponds to a variation within up to 1 standard deviation around the average and is considered a normal variation. Scores that exceed a deviation of 1.5 SD from the average may be taken as indicative of a deficit, and those that exceed 2 SD from the average should be taken with greater care, as there are stronger indications of a deficit (Fonseca et al., 2016).

To calculate the z-score, the professional will need the raw score (RS) obtained by their patient on a given instrument. Then, they should locate, in the manuals of the instruments used, the mean (M) and the standard deviation (SD) of the normative group that serves as a parameter for comparing his/her patient's performance. Then, just resort to a simple formula:

$$z = \frac{RS - M}{SD}$$

Once all raw scores are transformed into z-scores, they can be plotted on the same graph (as they are on the same scale). This action facilitates visual inspection and identification of a profile of skills and difficulties (weaknesses and strengths or "peaks" and "valleys"). Figure 1.1 illustrates this representation. On the x-axis are all the skills contemplated in the evaluation; the y-axis brings the score, already transformed into a z-score. The gray band is located between −1 and 1 SD (average performance range).

Given the profile presented in Fig. 1.1, consider the following complaint: *school difficulties, not understanding what he reads, and having problems even with simple addition. He always seems lost in tasks; one have to insist a lot so that he does his duties, and even then, he often stops halfway. He seems inattentive at times.*

The evaluation performed corroborates the complaint of difficulties at school. As word recognition skills and phonological awareness are preserved, another deficit is likely underlying the reading comprehension difficulties. The same reasoning applies to understanding difficulties in calculation since numerical processing is preserved. The skills profile shows short-term memory and linguistic skills preserved, as well as intelligence, but deficits in executive functions, more evident in working memory, followed by flexibility. There is ample evidence from the literature pointing to executive functions' role in reading comprehension and calculation. Thus, considering that pedagogical and socio-family conditions were adequate (aspects that should also be raised in the evaluation), a hypothesis would be

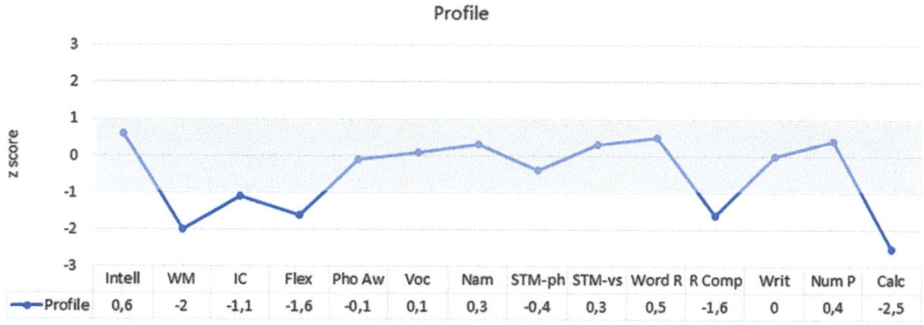

Fig. 1.1 Illustration of peaks and valleys profile from neuropsychological evaluation (***Intell*** **Intelligence,** ***WM*** **Working Memory,** ***IC*** **Inhibitory Control,** ***Flex*** **Cognitive Flexibility,** ***Pho Aw*** **Phonological Awareness,** ***Voc*** **Vocabulary,** ***Nam*** **Naming,** ***STM-ph*** **Short-term Phonological Memory,** ***STM-vs*** **Short-term Visuospatial Memory,** ***Word R*** **Word Recognition,** ***R Comp*** **Reading Comprehension,** ***Writ*** **Word Writing,** ***Num P*** **Numerical Processing,** ***Calc*** **Calculation)**

plausible that deficits in these skills could underlie the academic difficulties presented. The intervention would then have its initial targets defined.

In addition to planning the neuropsychological intervention, the evaluation also provides a whole range of knowledge about the case that allows for other directions, including necessary referrals to other professionals and guidance for those dealing with the child, such as teachers and parents. Such guidance, backed by knowledge of the patient's neuropsychological profile, will have a greater chance of being effective.

Final Considerations

To plan the intervention process (whether in habilitation or rehabilitation), it is essential to first identify the targets of this process. This role belongs to the neuropsychological evaluation, which allows for a detailed survey of the individual's cognitive, emotional, and behavioral difficulties and abilities, their context and interactions, as well as their daily functioning in performing activities. The articulation of this information allows us to understand how the impairments observed in the evaluation can impact their daily life and manifest in their behavior. This broad understanding is the initial and fundamental element of intervention planning. Here, the target skills of the process are defined, which allows us to think about the objectives to be achieved and, consequently, the stages and strategies of the intervention process. In short, the neuropsychological assessment fulfills the role of informing and directing the professional's intervention action.

Annex of Chapter

Anamnesis

(Model provided by Alessandra Gotuzo Seabra & Natália Martins Dias, based on Baron, 2004*)*

Date: / /

Contact phones:

Residential: Cell:

Street/Ave Neighborhood City

Identification

Full name:

Date of birth: / / Current Age: School Year:

School: private ( ) municipal ( ) state ( ) other ( ) _________

Name of the School: ____

Family data

Mother's name: ____

Date of birth / / Current Age:

Education: Occupation: ____

Father's name: ____

Date of birth / / Current Age:

Education: Occupation: ____

The parents are: married( ) separated( ) divorced( ) remarried ( ) other: _

If separated or divorced:

How old was the child at the time of separation? __________________________

Legal guardian of the child? ___________________________________

The child is: biological ( ) adopted ( )—at what age? ________ other: ________

Who currently lives with the child:

Name: ____

Relationship: ____

Age: ____

Initial Complaint

Tell us a little about why you are seeking this evaluation:

Describe your child's strengths:

Describe your child's areas of difficulty:

What is your child's routine DURING THE WEEK? (What time they wake up, what period they go to school, who they stay with when at home, favorite activities)

What is your child's routine ON THE WEEKEND? (What time they wake up, leisure activities, others)

Pregnancy and Birth History

At the child's birth: mother's age: ______________________ father's age: ______________________

Before this child, had the mother had any pregnancy: ______________________ or miscarriage: ______________________

During pregnancy, were there any medical complications?

During pregnancy, the mother:

Took medication? Yes( ) No( ) *If yes, which one?*

Smoked? Yes( ) No( ) *If yes, how many cigarettes per day?*

Drank alcohol? Yes( ) No( ) *If yes, how many drinks per day?*

Used drugs? Yes( ) No( ) *If yes, what type? How often?*

At how many weeks was the child born? ______________________

What type of birth? ______________________ How many hours of labor? ______________________

Birth weight: ________________________ Length: ________________________

Apgar: ____

Were there any complications at birth? (e.g., cord wrapped around the neck, lack of oxygen, and improper position of the baby)

Was there a need for medical intervention? (e.g., neonatal ICU, incubator, oxygenation)

How many days did the baby stay in the hospital?

Did the mother show any signs of postpartum depression?

How was the baby fed in the first few months?

How was the baby's sleep in the first few months?

Development

- **Motor**

  Age at which:

  Sat alone: _________ Crawled: _________ Stood alone: _________ Walked alone: _________

  Compared to other children of the same age, did your child seem different during development? (e.g., when running, jumping, playing ball, picking up objects, etc.) Explain:

Laterality: Right-handed ( ) Left-handed ( ) Ambidextrous ( ) Undefined ( )

In relation to children of the same age, does he/she seem:

more agitated ( ) similar motor behavior ( ) quieter ( )

Does the child currently confuse right and left? ___________________

Has the child ever had any type of motor therapy?

Has he/she practiced or does he/she practice sports? Which ones? What is the performance?

- **Linguistic**

  Age at which:

  Babbled: _____ Spoke the first word: ______ Spoke combinations of 2 to 3 words: ______

  Did the child seem to have any difficulty speaking? (stuttering, speech hard to understand):

Did the child have any other oral problem (drooled too much, poor suction etc.)?

Does the child have contact with any other language besides Portuguese? Explain.

How is the child's speech (organizes ideas well, has a good vocabulary, etc.)? Explain.

How is the child's understanding (does he/she understand well what is said to him/her)? Explain.

Does the child have a good memory of what is said to him/her?

Has the child ever had a speech therapy evaluation or therapy? If yes, why, at what age and for how long?

- **Toilet**

  Age at which toilet training began: ________________

  Age at which diapers were removed: daytime: ______________________ nighttime: ______________________

  Did the child have difficulties above the usual or did he/she wet the clothes or bed after toilet training?

Medical History

The child has had:

Vision exams: _____ Any problems? ____________________________________

Hearing exams: _____ Any problems? ____________________________________

Consultation with a neurologist? _______________ Reason: _______________
Any problems? _______________

Consultation with a psychiatrist? _______________ Reason: _______________
Any problems? _______________

Consultation with another medical specialist? ___________ Reason: ___________
Any problems?_______________

Mark the diseases the child has had and put the age:

() Otitis	() Fainting or loss of consciousness
() Sinusitis	() Paralysis
() Mumps	() Polio
() bronchitis	() Tonsillitis
() Meningitis or encephalitis	() Rubella
() Allergies	() Asthma
() Headaches	() Chickenpox
() Measles	() Whooping cough
() Abdominal pain/vomiting	() Heart problems
() Pneumonia	() Anemia
() Absences or epilepsy	() Diabetes
() Zika	() High blood pressure
() Yellow fever	() Poisoning
() Developmental regression	() Others: ________________

More serious diseases that required hospitalizations and ages at which they occurred:

____

____

____

Does the child take any medication? Why?

____

Is there a family history of any disease? If yes, who?

Physical ( )________________________ Psychiatric ( )____________________

Neurological ( )____________________ Epilepsy ( )______________________

Learning difficulties ( )______________ Attention difficulties ( )____________

Is there a history of drug use or alcohol abuse in the family? If yes, who?

____

Currently, how is the child's sleep?

( ) Sleeps well—how many hours per night? ______________________________

( ) Nightmares or difficulty sleeping

( ) Does not like to sleep alone

Does the child sleep in a room alone? If not, with whom? ___________________

What is their routine to fall asleep? ______________________________________

Currently, how is the child's eating?

( ) Eats poorly, has restricted diet or refuses to eat

( ) Overeats

( ) Has weight problems? Which? ______________________________________

Behavior

The child gets along with:
Other children of the same age? _________ Adults? _________.
Does they he/she have some good friends? ___________ Does he/she keep friends?
____________.

Did he/she like to be held or caressed as a baby? _________________.

Does he/she understand gestures? ____________ Does he/she have a good sense of humor? _____________.

Does he/she prefer to play alone or play with other people? (who?) _________________.

Does he/she understand social cues (notice when others are sad or angry)? ________.

He/she seems like a child:

Aggressive () Irritable () Shy () Stubborn () Affectionate ().

Worried () Nervous () Impulsive () Inattentive () Naive ().

Does the child seem to have difficulty with frustration?

Does he/she have difficulty in strange environments and situations?

Cognition

Compare your child's abilities with other children of the same age:

	Has difficulty	Is average	Has ease
Learns things outside of school			
Learns things at school			
Organizes well			
Maintains attention			
Remembers his/her commitments and duties			
Is intelligent			

Formal Learning

At what age did your child start school?

Was there any change of school? Explain.

Were there specific difficulties in any school year? Explain.

How did the child do in literacy?

How did he/she do in learning math?

Does the child like to read?

Does he/she swap letters or words when reading aloud?

Does he/she swap letters or words when writing?

Does he/she have difficulty in doing calculations or using money?

Does the teacher report any difficulty? Explain.

Was he/she recommended for tutoring (or school reinforcement)? In what year and subject?

Did he/she repeat any year?

Mark with an "X" in the subjects where he/she has more difficulty and ease.

	Has difficulty	Is average	Has ease
Language/reading			
Mathematics			
Science			
Geography			
History			
Physical education			
Foreign languages			
Arts			
Music			
Others: _______			

Neuropsychological History

Has the child ever had any other neuropsychological evaluation?

If yes, when and with which professional?

What were the results?

Other information you would like to add:

References

Associação Psiquiátrica Americana. (2014). *Manual Diagnóstico e Estatístico de Transtornos Mentais DSM-5*. Artmed.

Baron, I. S. (2004). *Neuropsychological evaluation of the child*. Oxford University Press.

Bosa, C. A., & Salles, J. F. (2018). *PROTEA-R Sistema de avaliação da suspeita de transtorno do espectro autista*. Vetor.

Cardoso, C. O., Dias, N. M., Seabra, A. G., & Fonseca, R. P. (2016). Processo de construção do programa de estimulação neuropsicológica de funções executivas e processos cognitivos relacionados em escolares. In C. O. Cardoso & R. P. Fonseca (Eds.), *Programa de Estimulação Neuropsicológica da Cognição em Escolares, com ênfase nas Funções Exeutivas*. Porto Alegre.

Costanzo, F., Varuzza, C., Menghini, D., Addona, F., Gianesini, T., & Vicari, S. (2013). Executive functions in intellectual disabilities: A comparison between Williams syndrome and Down syndrome. *Research in Developmental Disabilities, 34*(5), 1770–1780. https://doi.org/10.1016/J.RIDD.2013.01.024

Dias, N. M., & Seabra, A. G. (2013). *Programa de Intervenção em Autorregulação e Funções Executivas – PIAFEx*. Memnon.
Fonseca, R. P., Prando, M. L., & Zimmermann, N. (2016). *Tarefas para Avaliação Neuropsicológica: Avaliação de linguagem e funções executivas em crianças*. Memnon.
Freire, R. C. L., & Hazin, I. (2015). Perfil neuropsicológico e possibilidades de intervenção em sala de aula na Síndrome de Down. In N. M. Dias & T. P. Mecca (Eds.), *Contribuições da Neuropsicologia e Psicologia para intervenção no contexto educacional* (pp. 273–282). Memnon.
Hale, J. B., & Fiorello, C. A. (2004). *School neuropsychology: A practitioner's handbook*. Guilford Publications.
Major, S., & Seabra-Santos, M. J. (2013). Uso de inventários comportamentais para a avaliação socioemocional em idade pré-escolar. *Avaliação Psicológica, 12*(1), 101–107.
Major, S., & Seabra-santos, M. J. (2014). Pais e/ou Professores? Acordo entre Informadores na Avaliação Socioemocional de pré-escolares. *Psicologia: Teoria e Pesquisa, 30*(4), 373–383.
Malloy-Diniz, L. F., Haase, V. G., & Salles, J. F. (2017). *Neuropsicologia do Desenvolvimento*. Artmed.
Martoni, A. T., Trevisan, B. T., Dias, N. M., & Seabra, A. G. (2016). Funções executivas: relação entre relatos de pais, de professores e desempenho de crianças. *Temas em Psicologia, 24*(1), 173–188. https://doi.org/10.9788/TP2016.1-12
Miotto, E. (2016). O uso do exame neuropsicológico para estruturar uma intervenção. In L. F. Malloy-Diniz, P. Mattos, N. Abreu, & D. Fuentes (Eds.), *Neuropsicologia: aplicações clínicas* (pp. 209–222). Artmed.
Narzisi, A., Muratori, F., Calderoni, S., Fabbro, F., & Urgesi, C. (2013). Neuropsychological Profile in High Functioning Autism Spectrum Disorders. *Journal of Autism and Developmental Disorders, 43*(8), 1895–1909. https://doi.org/10.1007/s10803-012-1736-0
Neri, M. (2012). *Avaliação neuropsicológica de crianças com epilepsia rolândica*. Tese de Doutorado. Universidade Estadual de Campinas.
O'Brien, J. W., Dowell, L. R., Mostofsky, S. H., Denckla, M. B., & Mahone, E. M. (2010). Neuropsychological Profile of Executive Function in Girls with Attention-Deficit/Hyperactivity Disorder. *Archives of Clinical Neuropsychology, 25*(7), 656–670. https://doi.org/10.1093/arclin/acq050
Rueda, F. J. M., Noronha, A. P. P., Sisto, F. F., Santos, A. A. A., & Castro, N. R. (2013). *Escala Wechsler de Inteligência para Crianças–4ª Edição (WISC-IV): Manual Técnico*. Casa do Psicólogo.
Salles, J. F., Fonseca, R. P., Parente, M. A. M. P., Barbosa, T., Miranda, M. C., Cruz-Rodrigues, C., & Mello, C. B. (2016). *Instrumento de Avaliação Neuropsicológica Breve Infantil - NEUPSILIN-Inf*. Vetor.
Seabra, A. G., & Dias, N. M. (2012a). *Avaliação Neuropsicológica Cognitiva: atenção e funções executivas* (1st ed.). Memnon.
Seabra, A. G., & Dias, N. M. (2012b). *Avaliação Neuropsicológica Cognitiva: linguagem oral*. Memnon.
Seabra, A. G., Dias, N. M., & Macedo, E. C. (2012). Neuropsicologia cognitiva e avaliação neuropsicológica cognitiva: contexto, definição e objetivo. In A. G. Seabra & N. M. Dias (Eds.), *Avaliação Neuropsicológica Cognitiva: Atenção e funções executivas* (pp. 16–27). Memnon.
Seabra, A. G., Dias, N. M., & Capovilla, F. C. (2013). *Avaliação Neuropsicológica Cognitiva: leitura, escrita e aritmética*. Memnon.
Seabra-Santos, M. J., & Gaspar, M. F. F. (2012). Pais, educadores e testes: estão de acordo na avaliação de aptidões de crianças pré-escolares? *Psicologia: Reflexão e Crítica, 25*(2), 203–211. https://doi.org/10.1590/S0102-79722012000200001
Semrud-Clikeman, M., & Ellison, P. A. T. (2009). *Child Neuropsychology: Assessment and Intervention*. Springer.

Taylor, H. G., Dietrich, A., Nuss, K., Wright, M., Rusin, J., Bangert, B., Minich, N., & Yeates, K. O. (2010). Post-concussive symptoms in children with mild traumatic brain injury. *Neuropsychology, 24*(2), 148–159. https://doi.org/10.1037/a0018112

Thomson, J., Kerns, K., Seidenstrang, L., Sohlberg, M. M., & Mateer, C. (2017). *PAY ATTENTION! Programa de Intervenção dos Processos Atencionais para Crianças*. Hogrefe.

Toplak, M. E., West, R. F., & Stanovich, K. E. (2013). Practitioner review: Do performance-based measures and ratings of executive function assess the same construct? *Journal of Child Psychology and Psychiatry, 54*(2), 131–143. https://doi.org/10.1111/jcpp.12001

Uzzell, B. P., Ponton, M., & Ardila, A. (2013). *International handbook of cross-cultural neuropsychology*. Psychology Press.

Chapter 2
Child Neuropsychological Intervention

Caroline de Oliveira Cardoso and Rochele Paz Fonseca

Neuropsychological intervention is internationally better known under the term neuropsychological rehabilitation. However, there are several objectives to intervene in one or more cognitive domains in favor of more efficient cognitive performance and functionality of an individual in everyday life. Regarding the demands of child neurodevelopment, there are objectives of prevention and stimulation as early as possible.

Traditionally, neuropsychological rehabilitation corresponds to a complex set of procedures and techniques to improve or enhance cognitive, behavioral, and emotional processes, allowing the patient a better quality of life. After the process of neuropsychological evaluation, in which the cognitive profile of the patient (skills and difficulties) is identified and the impact of deficits on their functionality is understood, many professionals ask themselves: *Given this mapping of better developed/preserved cognitive skills and less developed/impaired/deficient cognitive skills, what do I do? How can I help my patient improve their performance and functionality?* In this chapter, initially, the general principles and the main approaches of neuropsychological rehabilitation will be presented. Then, the focus will be on neuropsychological interventions with children. Although, historically, child rehabilitation was based on adult rehabilitation, its peculiarities and differences are recognized today. With this, throughout the chapter, these points will be discussed and some particular models for children will be presented.

C. O. Cardoso (✉)
Universidade Feevale, Novo Hamburgo, Rio Grande do Sul, Brazil
e-mail: carolinecardoso@feevale.br

R. P. Fonseca
Universidade Federal de Minas Gerais, Belo Horizonte, Conectare Neuropsi, Brazil
e-mail: rochele.fonseca@gmail.com

C. O. Cardoso, N. M. Dias (eds.), *Neuropsychological Interventions for Children - Volume 1*, https://doi.org/10.1007/978-3-031-53586-4_2

Neuropsychological Rehabilitation

Neuropsychological rehabilitation is the treatment approach to improve impaired cognitive processes and/or adapt the patient to acquired deficits, aiming at the highest level of possible adaptation and better quality of life. Wilson (1989, 2008) defines it as a process in which people with brain damage work with health professionals, family members, and community members to remedy or minimize cognitive deficits. It is worth noting that for many years neuropsychological rehabilitation was restricted to patients with acquired injuries. However, currently there are several programs and interventions aimed both at patients who present some cognitive dysfunction (examples: children who present neurodevelopmental disorder, such as Attention Deficit Hyperactivity Disorder, Autism Spectrum Disorder) as well as interventions aimed at stimulating cognitive skills early and preventively. Throughout the chapter, different intervention modalities will be presented and discussed.

In the literature, there are various terms to define this type of intervention, the most common being cognitive rehabilitation, cognitive training and neuropsychological rehabilitation (Cicerone et al., 2011; Wilson, 2008; Wilson et al., 2017). It is possible to make a differentiation, although they are often used as synonyms (Gindri et al., 2012). Cognitive rehabilitation describes interventions or techniques that assist in improving cognitive deficits caused by injuries or dysfunctions, aiming to stimulate cognitive functions altered through cognitive training (Ciccerone et al., 2011; Grindi et al., 2012; Wilson, 2008). On the other hand, the term neuropsychological rehabilitation is broader since, in addition to seeking to improve cognitive deficits, it emphasizes the emotional, psychosocial, and behavioral aspects of a brain injury or dysfunction (Grindi et al., 2012; Wilson, 2008). Thus, it is noted that the term neuropsychological rehabilitation is associated with a more global, holistic approach to intervention.

From a historical point of view, there has been interest in cognitive rehabilitation since antiquity. However, the first systematic procedures only emerged during the First and Second World Wars, a period in which there was a significant increase in demand for adult rehabilitation due to surviving soldiers with brain injuries. During this period, health professionals sought to understand how the different types of injury influenced human behavior and how to intervene to remedy these cognitive deficits (Poser, 1996; Wilson, 2008). Doctors joined educators to develop, together, methods of "relearning." Although many concepts remain, there have been important changes in the field of rehabilitation, especially in the 1990s, considered the decade of the brain (Baddeley et al., 2000), when there was a greater understanding and definition of approaches. Among the major changes, the need for goal definition for neuropsychological rehabilitation planning stands out, the need for different theoretical models to support rehabilitation and, with the advancement of programs, it was possible to propose a classification considering the method of interventions (Wilson, 2008).

Wilson (1997), when discussing the state of the art of cognitive rehabilitation, mentions four main approaches: (1) based on cognitive training through exercises, (2) based on models of cognitive neuropsychology, (3) combined approach (models derived from neuropsychology, cognitive psychology, and behavioral psychology), and (4) holistic approach.

In **cognitive training**, the aim is to recover or improve cognitive skills using specific exercises or cognitive training. For this, various strategies of repetition and structured practice of tasks are used. Wilson (1997) points out that the focus is on cognitive impairment, not on disabilities and difficulties brought about by cognitive deficits. Furthermore, it is considered a disadvantage that it is directed toward the progress of cognitive performance and by the absence of secure evidence of the treatment effect (Abrisqueta-Gomez & Silva, 2017).

The **cognitive neuropsychology approach** initially involves conducting a neuropsychological assessment to identify cognitive impairments and understand the nature of the problem so that, at a second moment, an intervention based on cognitive training can be proposed. The patient's progress is verified in the performance of the trained task and in the neuropsychological reassessment (Abrisqueta-Gomes & Silva, 2017; Wilson, 1997).

The **combined approach** involves various areas, disciplines and models derived from cognitive neuropsychology, behavioral psychology and learning theory, among others, to work with the patient on the consequences of a brain injury. However, this approach still cannot accommodate emotional problems, such as self-awareness and psychosocial adjustments of patients (Abrisqueta-Gomez & Silva, 2017; Wilson, 1997).

Finally, the **holistic approach,** initially developed by Diller (1976), Ben-Yishay (1978), Prigatano (1986) and Wilson (2002), is one of the most used models today. This approach seeks to work on cognitive components and the emotional and psychosocial aspects of brain injuries or dysfunctions. It is considered that personality components and emotional state can interfere in the rehabilitation process. Therefore, it uses awareness of the patient's deficits, as well as the possibility of incorporating psychotherapy into the rehabilitation process. In this approach, the objectives are functional and with goals related to real life. Thus, generalization and transfer of gains from the clinical setting to everyday cognitive demands are advocated.

In cases of neuropsychological rehabilitation with children, it is still more common to find in the literature cognitive training based on stimulation of an isolated cognitive function through exercises and well-defined activities using concrete materials or computerized activities (Barbosa, 2011; Sant'Anna & Mello, 2017). However, some studies propose holistic neuropsychological rehabilitation for children (Marcantuono & Prigatano, 2008; Sant'Anna & Mello, 2017). Throughout the chapter, holistic interventions will be presented in greater detail.

In summary, it is possible to highlight that, in the current view, the role of neuropsychological rehabilitation is not simply limited to the remediation of cognitive deficits through systematic training. Neuropsychological rehabilitation also encompasses the interest in working and addressing the emotional and behavioral aspects associated with brain injuries and dysfunctions. Although it is possible to classify interventions, it is important to note that the methods are not mutually exclusive, being quite common the use of cognitive training and the holistic approach during the rehabilitation process, the first for its specificity and the second, consequently, for its greater potential for generalization to real life. The patient's demands, goals, and individual factors, such as age and cognitive and emotional functioning, will indicate the method(s) adopted by the professional.

Neuropsychological Interventions in Childhood: Definitions, Objectives, and Particularities

The objectives of child neuropsychological rehabilitation are similar to the general intervention process with adults. It is an intervention in which the therapist works with the child, their family and the school to compensate, restore or enhance cognitive and behavioral processes. In the literal sense, rehabilitation refers to the return to some level of the previous state, restoring a previous condition. Thus, such a term can generate confusion for many professionals and for the patient and their relatives (Covre, 2017), especially for children, where many cognitive deficits do not arise due to a neurological condition but rather a neurodevelopmental disorder.

With this, there is a proposal to use the following nomenclatures depending on the neurological condition (structural or functional) and the objective of rehabilitation (preventive or remedial), as seen in Fig. 2.1. When the intervention involves rehabilitating, remedying cognitive processes that were impaired after brain injury, the suggested term is **rehabilitation**. In situations where cognitive deficits do not arise as a result of a neurological condition but are more associated with less opportunity for natural cognitive stimulation or developmental changes, the intervention process is called **habilitation**. From the perspective of neuropsychology, in habilitation, usually related to children with neurodevelopmental disorders, it is proposed to assist in the acquisition and development of skills that have not yet been acquired by the individual or that are performing below in their daily tasks in relation to the

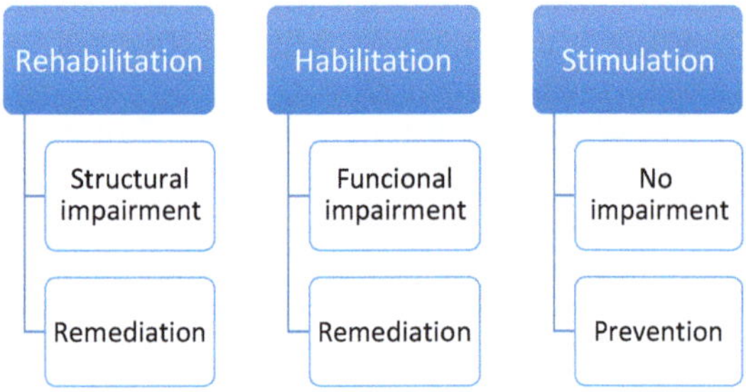

Fig. 2.1 Classification of neuropsychological interventions

demand of the environment. Both rehabilitation and habilitation are remedial interventions. There are also interventions to promote cognitive stimulation in periods a little before or at the time when optimal development windows are expected to be open, called **early-preventive interventions.**

Regarding children, caveats need to be made, and some particularities in relation to adulthood should be considered. Children's brains are in the process of maturation and, with this, cognitive processes are developing. Brain maturation is a complex phenomenon involving various aspects, such as genetic, structural, and neuroplasticity (Miranda et al., 2018). There is no single model that allows identifying at what age and in what order the different cognitive processes reach maturity (Crone & Ridderinkhof, 2011; Rajeswaran et al., 2013). In complementarity, neuroimaging studies show that the brain structures recruited to perform cognitive tasks change with age. For example, adults recruit the dorsolateral prefrontal region and parietal cortex in a visuospatial working memory activity. At the same time, children activate the regions of the caudate nucleus and the anterior insula more (Scherf et al., 2006). In addition, neuropsychological dysfunctions in childhood have much more heterogeneous characteristics than homogeneous, precisely because of the various possible developmental trajectories (greater individual variability). All these points make child neuropsychological intervention quite challenging.

Children who have acquired injury, such as from traumatic brain injury, meningitis or stroke, may present significant cognitive impairments and behavioral changes. Despite the child's brain being more plastic than the adult's and being more susceptible to recovery from an injury, it is known that the earlier the injury, the more difficult the recovery tends to be, as more complex cognitive subprocesses depend on more basic neurocognitive domains that, the earlier the injury occurs, the more impaired they will be. This means that the younger the child has an acquired injury, especially diffuse or generalized injuries, the less stock (or reserve) of skills they have, which increases the possibility of greater cognitive impairment. As the brain regions are still in the process of maturation and the functions are not clearly defined, early brain injuries can generate greater difficulties in acquiring basic skills necessary for development (Rajeswaran et al., 2013). However, it is important to emphasize that the earlier the detection and intervention, the greater the benefits and the better the prognosis.

In this way, the child's age is an important variable for planning the intervention. In cognitive terms, it is always important to consider what is expected for each age group to provide appropriate interventions for each case. Moreover, it is known that the child's education, as well as the parents' education (Ardila et al., 2005), type of school (Casarin et al., 2012) and socioeconomic level (Farah et al., 2006; Piccolo et al., 2014) are also variables that need to be considered, as they directly influence cognitive development. Sociocultural factors interact with individuals, such as age, and can stimulate positive neuroplasticity (generating more effective connections with better resulting cognitive strategies) or negative neuroplasticity (fewer effective connections with less successful strategies).

Another point that differs from rehabilitation with adults is the presence and the need for parental participation. In adult rehabilitation, the family is also important;

however, when it comes to children dependent on their caregivers, the family assumes an even more relevant role (Santos, 2005). Studies show that when the family is present, it helps the child improve their skills, supporting and encouraging them, managing to bring significant benefits to the child's behavioral and emotional functioning (Taylor et al., 2002; Yeates et al., 2010). For parents to be able to encourage and help their children, the therapist needs to provide support to the family. Thus, it is important that, during the rehabilitation process, a moment of welcoming the parents is provided so they can express how they have been feeling (guilt, anger, sadness, mourning for the loss, denial) and their concerns. It is also necessary to provide a moment of parental psychoeducation, which aims to teach parents about the etiology of the disease, about the skills and the cognitive difficulties of their child, as well as to teach strategies for them to stimulate the child. Due to these new responsibilities, the family needs to be prepared and enabled by the therapist to better assist in the child's recovery.

In addition to the family, the presence of the school is also relevant in this context; just like the parents, the teachers need to receive support. Given the results obtained in the neuropsychological evaluation, the teachers need to be psychoeducated about the brain injury or dysfunction and the student's cognitive abilities and difficulties associated with neurological factors as well as factors associated with parental characteristics and/or school characteristics or the life history of their student(s). With this information, the teacher, in conjunction with the therapist, understands the student's particular needs and can make some changes. In many cases, a major to minor adaptation, or curricular facilitation, is necessary.

Another aspect that is different from rehabilitation with adults is the environment and use of playful stimuli during rehabilitation. Before starting treatment, it is recommended that the therapist knows each child's preferences. For example, they can conduct a semi-structured questionnaire to learn about the child's favorite games, television programs, children's cartoons, and books, as well as the extracurricular activities they participate in (soccer, ballet, judo). Knowledge of preference for specific visual, auditory, olfactory, gustatory and olfactory stimuli is essential for the design of stimulation tasks. Given this information, you can create stimuli with the child's preferred themes. It is believed that by respecting the playful nature and using games and activities that the child identifies with, there can be an increase in the motivational level, generating greater engagement and collaboration. In addition, greater external transfer (generalization) from the neuropsychological *setting* to the home tends to occur.

In this perspective, Hunter and Donders (2007) proposed eight key concepts that we should consider when planning a child intervention:

1. Suitability to the level of development, that is, planning and conducting activities suitable for the typical cognitive repertoire of the child's development phase;
2. Orientation toward functionality to improve real-life performance;
3. Customization for an individualized plan, based on understanding complaints and results obtained in the neuropsychological evaluation, also considering the child's interests and preferences;

4. Developmental or longitudinal characteristics: it is known that childhood disorders change over time and with age. Therefore, it is important to set goals to prevent or minimize future problems;
5. Based on knowledge of cognitive systems;
6. Central pillar in the family, establishing a strong partnership with family members;
7. Transdisciplinarity, with cooperation among all professionals involved in the child's follow-up; and.
8. Scientificity, creating clear goals that can be measured.

Neuropsychological Re(h)abilitation

Before any re(h)abilitation process, it is essential to identify, from the neuropsychological evaluation, the difficulties and cognitive, emotional, and behavioral skills of the individual and understand how these impairments affect their daily lives. Only after this process does the re(h)abilitation begin. The first step in re(h)abilitation is planning and setting goals. Each treatment is individualized and planned based on deficits, skills, and environmental aspects in which the child is inserted. Therefore, there is no guide or a one-size-fits-all recipe.

One way to plan re(h)abilitation is based on health and disease models that allow a logical and systematic analysis of clinical problems. The International Classification of Functioning (ICF), developed by the World Health Organization (WHO, 2001), corresponds to an international system that classifies states, conditions, and causes of health problems and has been widely used to define the therapeutic planning of the health team (Palisano, 2006) and to facilitate communication among professionals (Andrade et al., 2009; Battistella & Brito, 2002). In Brazil, some studies propose the use of the ICF for planning rehabilitation in children (Andrade et al., 2009; Oliveira, 2014). In general, the ICF exposes functionality and disability due to disease and seeks to understand the relationship between the deficiencies in body structures and functions and psychosocial factors (environment and personal) and the activities and participation of the patient. From this, it is possible to extract information about the functionality and disability of the individual, making the target problems that need to be worked on more evident.

After filling out the ICF, the goals are set. The goals will guide the entire re(h)abilitation program. It is important to emphasize that they need to be individualized, patient-centered, defined in conjunction with family members and other involved professionals and aimed at improving the patient's functionality and quality of life. In this sense, some rehabilitation centers use the SMART system (from the acronym: S—*specific*, M—*measurable*, A—*achievable*, R—*relevant*, T—*timed*). According to this system, the goals must be specific, measurable, achievable, and relevant and have a set time. For example, for a patient with organizational difficulties, the goal "improve the ability to organize daily life" is too vague, and it is hard to identify fulfillment and may be unachievable. Additionally, setting a goal to "use the agenda to plan your daily routine" can also be considered inadequate, as the agenda may correspond to an intervention strategy. On the other hand, the goal "increase the ability to organize to deliver homework" is a specific goal; patients and family will know where they intend to go, and we can know if we achieved it or not.

Setting goals is not always simple; however, when well established, they allow the professional to better develop their strategies to achieve it, as much as it allows to evaluate the effectiveness of the intervention (Covre, 2017; Wilson et al., 2009). It can also motivate those involved, directing their focus and effort (Wada, 2009).

Once the goals are established, the therapist develops strategies that will be used to achieve them and, with this, a treatment plan is assembled. At this stage, it determines which strategies and techniques will be used, the frequency of training, and how behavior will be recorded (Nery-Barbosa & Barbosa, 2017). At this point, the professional can combine different strategies and techniques. For example, to increase the ability to organize for homework delivery, the clinician can propose cognitive training to improve organization and planning skills, propose environmental modification, with the organization of a routine or inclusion of a calendar, can guide parents on how to help their child in this task, offering positive reinforcements when the activity is performed as agreed. Mcmillan and Greenwood (1993) emphasize that neuropsychological rehabilitation should navigate the fields of clinical neuropsychology, behavioral analysis, cognitive training, and individual and group psychotherapy. Some techniques will be discussed below.

- ***Psychoeducation***—This technique aims to educate patients and family members about difficulties and skills, the course of the disease, and the form of treatment to provide greater awareness and acceptance of deficits (Gindri et al., 2012). Different materials, such as pamphlets, books, films, etc., can be used for this. Some tools are available in child rehabilitation, such as the book for children with specific learning disorders "Paul and the difficult task of learning to read—understanding dyslexia" (Bortoncello & Moraes, 2017).
- ***Restoration or enablement of cognitive function through training***—This technique aims to "train" cognitive functions and generate new learnings through specific exercises. However, it is emphasized that proposing several exercises without organization and purpose will possibly not generate generalization and transfer to everyday life. The approach based on trial and error attempts is neither ethical nor scientifically based. Thus, before starting games and exercises, it is recommended that psychoeducation and metacognitive training be carried out with the child to explain the cognitive function target of stimulation and where, how and why to use the strategies that will be taught. Creating a playful context using narratives, books, films or puppets is recommended. In this way, it is possible that there is greater engagement on the part of the patient since visual images and children's stories allow the child to develop better mnemonic and emotional connections (Cardoso & Fonseca, 2016). In addition, the mediation of language and real communicative demand provide verbal context and generally make activities more complex as in everyday social and school situations.

After psychoeducation, the professional seeks to stimulate the target cognitive function using games, exercises and playful materials. For this, public knowledge games can be used (UNO, LINCE, PASSWORD, memory, general with dice, dominos, various board and computerized games...), and pencil and paper activities or activities available on the internet. When developing or opting for some activities, it is important that the resources are used sequentially, repeated a few times, and that gradually, the level of difficulty and complexity increases (starting with easier tasks to more complex ones). After completing each activity, the professional can provide *feedback* on the performance and progress of the patient and help the child reflect on what was worked on through questions and inquiries. By providing this reflective environment, the therapist allows the patient to transfer what they learned to everyday situations, in addition to stimulating the development of self-knowledge and metacognition.

Currently, a wide variety of programs and digital games are available on websites (for example, Our Daily Brain, Lumosity). However, many of these programs do not have evidence of effectiveness and transfer analysis to functionality. One of the computerized programs that has studies showing its effectiveness (Klingberg et al., 2005; Thorell et al., 2009) is the Cogmed Working Memory Training, commercially available. It is an online training with versions for both preschoolers and school-age children. However, transfer studies are still inconclusive, as they seem not to favor the transfer of gains to other areas and situations (Melby-Lervåg et al., 2016).

Another example is Pay Attention! (Thomson et al., 2005), which was developed for children aged 4–14 years to stimulate sustained, selective, alternate, and divided attention and is also available in Brazil (Barbosa et al., 2014). There is also specific software developed in Brazil aimed at stimulating auditory skills (Pedro in the haunted house) (Santos et al., 2006), phonological awareness (Pedro in the amusement park) (Santos et al., 2008) and neurocognitive functions in a more global way (Pedro at the Camp) (Santos et al., 2012). Pedro at the Camp, for example, consists of ten games aimed at improving cognitive skills, such as attention, perception, executive functions, and oral and written language. It is suitable for children from 5 years old. Also noteworthy is the Neuropsychological Stimulation Program of Cognition in School Children with emphasis on executive functions (PENcE) (Cardoso & Fonseca, 2016), which was originally developed to stimulate executive functions in the school environment in elementary school children, with a version to use in the clinical environment (Rysdyk et al., 2016). It is important to reiterate that implementing these programs in isolation is insufficient to stimulate cognitive functions and generate improvements in daily life. Hence, it is important to integrate various strategies. In section "Neuropsychological interventions in childhood: Definitions, objectives and particularities" of this book, activity proposals and programs to stimulate attention (Chap. 7), memory (Chap. 8), executive functions (Chap. 9), theory of mind (Chap. 10), socio-emotional skills (Chap. 11), and school skills (Chaps. 12 and 13) will be presented.

- ***Compensatory strategies***—They are alternative strategies that help children compensate for their cognitive difficulties to reduce the functional impact of cognitive impairments. Examples of compensatory strategies include using a diary or calendar to organize and note school and social commitments. In school, for example, more time may be provided for the activity when it comes to a child with attentional or processing speed difficulties.
- ***Environment adaptation***—Management of stimuli and environmental dynamics can be very useful to optimize other interventions or as the main intervention itself, as environmental variables greatly interfere in the relationship between the cognitive offer of each case and the environmental demand for cognition. These are modifications of the physical environment to minimize distractors in the place, organize the space and adapt it to each patient's demand, aiming to reduce the patient's functional deficits (Nery-Barbosa & Barbosa, 2017). For example, when a child has difficulty with attention and concentration, it may be proposed to reduce the number of objects in the place, specifying the space where they will perform school tasks in the absence of stimuli such as television, video games, computer; include a whiteboard in the room so it can be used for studies and to note priorities or tasks for the day or week; acquire folders or files for the child to use to organize their materials, such as tests and assignments.
- ***Behavioral techniques***—In addition to cognitive difficulties, many children may present behavioral and emotional problems, and rehabilitation can also integrate intervention aimed at these problems. Currently, the interface of neuropsychology and behavior analysis is being proposed. Behavior analysis contributes with its procedures for promoting learning and behavioral changes. It offers the neuropsychologist tools to perform contingency analysis and greater knowledge of behavioral techniques (modeling, extinction, reinforcement, *role-playing*) (Pontes & Hubner, 2008). For example, when a desired behavior is not in the child's repertoire, we can use the technique of modeling and verbal instruction; when we want to maintain or increase a behavior, positive reinforcement or token economy[1] can be techniques used; in turn, to decrease or reduce problematic behavior, one can make use of the extinction technique, which consists of suppressing the reinforcement of a previously reinforced behavior. To use these techniques, it is fundamental, beforehand, to perform a functional analysis of the behavior, aiming to understand the environmental contingencies. That is, it seeks to identify the inappropriate behavior, the events that precede it, the environmental conditions that maintain it and the effect of the behavior on the environment, understanding the controlled variables and maintainers of behavior. With this analysis, the focus of the intervention and the most appropriate techniques for the patient become clear (Lopes & Dalmaso, 2017). If, for example, the antecedent factors are influencing the behavior, procedures that modify the antecedent stimuli (for example, modeling and *fading*) can be employed; if the consequent factors are the determinants, techniques that modify the consequents can be used (for example, establishment of reinforcement schemes) (Pontes & Hubner, 2008).

[1] Systematic reinforcement program in which points or tokens are awarded each time the patient presents the desired behavior.

Table 2.1 Examples of how to structure the planning of neuropsychological re/habilitation

Problem	Goal	Explanatory hypotheses	Strategies
Interrupts others' conversations and does not wait their turn to speak	Decrease interruption in peers' conversations and wait their turn to speak	Inhibitory Control	Psychoeducate the child, teaching the Stop, Think and Follow strategy, with the traffic light metaphor; Psychoeducate parents and school and teach strategy and request that they give *feedback* to the child; Games and activities that stimulate inhibitory control; Behavioral techniques, such as token economy.
Does not concentrate on activities, especially when doing school tasks	Being able to concentrate on doing school activities	Selective attention and inhibitory control	Psychoeducate the child, parents, and school about the behavior that is desired to change; Propose modifications in the environment—change the time to do the tasks, establish a routine, appropriate place, without many stimuli, take more frequent breaks when performing the tasks; Games and activities that stimulate selective attention and inhibitory control.

Below, in Table 2.1, some examples of the planning of a child neuropsychological rehabilitation are provided, in which the goals were set, the explanatory hypothesis was raised and some strategies were listed.

Early-Preventive Neuropsychological Stimulation

In neuropsychology, actions and interventions are mainly directed at patients with some brain injury or cognitive dysfunction, with the main purpose of evaluating and remedying/treating the effects caused by such disorders, thus configuring a tertiary level of prevention (Wilson, 2008). However, currently, many researchers and professionals in the health and education fields are increasingly interested in interventions aimed at stimulating, improving, and enhancing skills without accelerating, but rather trying to ensure the optimal development expected for each age group, being considered an intervention at the primary level of neuropsychological health care. This type of intervention can also play an important preventive role in the sense that it is planned to be used with children in typical development to enhance cognitive processes and avoid future damage.

In a systematic review of the literature, Cardoso et al. (2016) found 19 studies. Generally, it was possible to verify that cognitive skills, specifically executive

Table 2.2 Modalities of early-preventive neuropsychological intervention

Characteristics	Computerized training	Curriculum adaptation	Metacognitive approach
Modality	Individual.	Group.	Group or Individual.
Mediation	Professional.	Teacher.	Teacher.
Task format	Stimulates specific components—specific tasks.	Stimulation of self-regulation—global tasks.	Stimulation of metacognition—involves teaching to monitor and manage own skills.
Advantages	Attractive programs, generates motivation in the participant. Automatically increases the level of difficulty of the tasks.	More generalizable gains and in functionality. Improvement of academic skills and generates behavioral changes. Little investment required.	Proposes systematic strategies on how to teach cognitive skills to children.
Disadvantages	Relatively high economic investment for schools (license per student). Controversial findings regarding transfer effect.	Difficult to determine the relationship between activities and the stimulated cognitive component, because the tasks are broader and more global.	There is no systematic program with effectiveness analysis; there are tips and guidelines.

functions, can be developed and enhanced in children through systematic interventions. This study also showed that this intervention usually occurs in the school context since it is an environment with a significant number of children in typical development. In addition, considering the modality of the programs, it is possible to classify whether the intervention is a (1) computerized cognitive training, (2) curriculum adaptation or (3) instruction of cognitive strategies/metacognitive approach (Cardoso et al., 2016; Otero et al., 2014). In Table 2.2 it is possible to better understand each of these modalities, considering structure, mediator, task format, advantages, and disadvantages.

Final Considerations

As mentioned throughout the chapter, the process of neuropsychological intervention can be classified depending on the neurological condition (structural or functional) and the objective of the intervention (preventive or remedial) into neuropsychological rehabilitation, neuropsychological habilitation, and early-preventive neuropsychological intervention. Regardless of the modality, child neuropsychological intervention is still a recent field of action and with little scientific research. However, there is already evidence that cognitive training in isolation (non-holistic approach) has predominantly effects with proximal transfer in tasks very similar to those that were trained. The more holistic and ecological approach, in which there is an approximation with the demands of the patient's daily life, in addition to demonstrating a proximal transfer effect, there is evidence of improvement and gains in functionality, with improvement in school performance and emotional aspects.

When it comes to interventions with children, in addition to the construction of a detailed intervention plan with the goals, strategies, and techniques that will be used, it is essential that there is a partnership between therapist, patient, family, and school. It is known that the engagement of the family and school, in conjunction with strategies adopted by the professional, will allow the intervention to succeed.

From future perspectives, in addition to the need for greater investment in research, from case studies to controlled trials, there is also the need to invest in evaluative tasks for intervention outcomes, both cognitive functionality of the necessary subdomains in daily life (inventories, scales), as well as in outcome measures for intervention. In addition, it is important to increasingly standardize programs with their records, that is, to check what is expected of evolution from each session for each age group and educational level, and at the end of each module, for example.

References

Abrisqueta-Gomez, J., & Silva, K. K. M. (2017). Fundamentos da reabilitação cognitiva. In L. Malloy-Diniz, P. Mattos, N. Abreu, & D. Fuentes (Eds.), *Neuropsicologia aplicações clínicas* (pp. 223–241). Artmed.

Andrade, P. M. O., Ferreira, F. O., & Haase, V. G. (2009). Classificação Internacional de Funcionalidade, Incapacidade e Saúde (CIF) e o trabalho interdisciplinar no Sistema Único de Saúde (SUS). In V. G. Haase, F. O. Ferreira, & F. Penna (Eds.), *O enfoque biopsicossocial à saúde da criança e do adolescente* (pp. 67–88). COOPMED.

Ardila, A., Rosselli, M., Matute, E., & Guajardo, S. (2005). The influence of the parents educational level on the development of executive functions. *Developmental Neuropsychology, 28*(1), 539–560.

Arruda, M. A., Pinheiro, C. Q., Barros, C., Mata, M. F., Rezende, G., & Arroyo, L. H. (2015). *Cartilha do Terapeuta. Método Glia*. Ed. Instituto Glia.

Baddeley, A., Bueno, O., Cahill, L., Fuster, J. M., Izquierdo, I., Mcgaugh, J. L., Morris, R. G. M., Nadel, L., Routtenberg, A., Xavier, G., & da Cunha, C. (2000). The brain decade in debate: I. Neurobiology of learning and memory. *Brazilian Journal of Medical and Biological Research, 33*, 993–1002.

Barbosa, D. L. F. (2011). *Reabilitação cognitiva da atenção: tradução e adaptação do Pay Attention! A children's attention process training program* (Dissertação de Mestrado, Unifesp).

Barbosa, D. L. F., Miranda, M. C., & Bueno, O. F. A. (2014). Tradução e Adaptação do Pay Attention!–Um Programa de Treinamento dos Processos da Atenção para Crianças. *Psicologia: Reflexão e Crítica, 27*(4), 775–783. https://doi.org/10.1590/1678-7153.201427418

Battistella, L. R., & Brito, C. M. M. (2002). Tendência e Reflexões: Classificação Internacional de Funcionalidade (CIF). *Acta Fisiátrica, 9*(2), 98–101.

Ben-Yishay, Y. (1978). *Working approaches to remediation of cognitive deficits in brain damaged persons (Rehabilitation Monograph No. 59)*. New York University Medical Center.

Bortoncello, C., & Moraes, D. S. F. (2017). *Paulo e a difícil tarefa de aprender a ler: compreendendo a dislexia*. Sinopsys Editora.

Cardoso, C. O., & Fonseca, R. P. (2016). *Programa de Estimulação Neuropsicológica da Cognição em Escolares: ênfase nas Funções Executivas*. BookToy.

Cardoso, C. O., Dias, N. M., Senger, J., Colling, A. P. C., Seabra, A. G., & Fonseca, R. P. (2016). Neuropsychological stimulation of executive functions in children with typical development: A systematic review. *Applied Neuropsychology: Child, 7*(1), 61–81. https://doi.org/10.1080/21622965.2016.1241950

Casarin, F. S., Wong, C. E. I., Parente, M. A. M. P., Salles, J. F., & Fonseca, R. P. (2012). Comparison of neuropsychological performance between students from public and private Brazilian schools. *Spanish Journal of Psychology, 15*(3), 942–951. https://doi.org/10.5209/rev_SJOP.2012.v15.n3.39386

Cicerone, K. D., Langenbahn, D. M., Braden, C., Malec, J. F., Kalmar, K., Fraas, M., Felicetti, T., Laatsch, L., Harley, J. P., Bergguist, T., Azulay, J., Cantor, J., & Ashman, T. (2011). Evidence-based cognitive rehabilitation: Updated review of the literature from 2003 through 2008. *Archives of Physical Medicine and Rehabilitation, 92*(4), 519–530. https://doi.org/10.1016/j.apmr.2010.11.015

Covre, P. (2017). O processo do estabelecimento de metas em reabilitação neuropsicológica. In D. R. Fontoura, L. Tisser, O. Bueno, S. Bolognani, & T. Frison (Eds.), *Teoria e prática na reabilitação neuropsicológica* (pp. 69–80). Vetor.

Crone, E. A., & Ridderinkhof, K. R. (2011). The developing brain: From theory to neuroimaging and back. *Developmental Cognitive Neuroscience, 1*, 101–109. https://doi.org/10.1016/j.dcn.2010.12.001

Diller, L. (1976). A model for cognitive retraining in rehabilitation. *The Clinical Psychologist, 26*, 13–15.

Farah, M. J., Shera, D. M., Savage, J. H., Betancourt, L., Giannetta, J. M., Brodsky, N. L., Malmud, E. K., & Hurt, H. (2006). Childhood poverty: Specific associations with neurocognitive development. *Brain Research, 1110*, 166–174. https://doi.org/10.1016/j.brainres.2006.06.072

Gindri, G., Frison, T. B., Oliveira, C. R., Zimmermann, N., Netto, T. M., Landeira-Fernandez, J., Parente, M. A. M. P., Ferré, P., Joanett, Y., & Fonseca, R. P. (2012). Métodos em reabilitação neuropsicológica. In J. Landeira-Fernandez & S. S. Fukusima (Eds.), *Métodos em neurociência* (pp. 343–375). Manole.

Hunter, S. J., & Donders, J. (2007). *Pediatric neuropsychological intervention*. Cambridge University Press.

Klingberg, T., Fernell, E., Olesen, P. J., Johnson, M., Gustafsson, P., Dahlström, K., Gillberg, C. G., Forssberg, H., & Westerberg, H. (2005). Computerized training of working memory in children with ADHD-A randomized, controlled trial. *Journal of the American Academy of Child & Adolescent Psychiatry, 44*(2), 177–186. https://doi.org/10.1097/00004583-200502000-00010

Lopes, K. V., & Dalmoso, B. (2017). Procedimentos de intervencao em neuropsicologia baseados na análise do comportamento. In L. Malloy-Diniz, P. Mattos, N. Abreu, & D. Fuentes (Eds.), *Neuropsicologia aplicações clinicas* (pp. 242–254). Artmed.

Marcantuono, J. T., & Prigatano, G. P. (2008). A holistic brain injury rehabilitation program for school-age children. *NeuroRehabilitation, 23*, 457–466.

McMillan, T. M., & Greenwood, R. J. (1993). Model of rehabilitation programmer for the brain-injured adult—Model services and suggestions for chance in the UK. *Clinical Rehabilitation, 6*, 346–355.

Melby-Lervag, M., Redick, T. S., & Hulme, C. (2016). Working memory training does not improve performance on measures of intelligence or other measures of "far transfer"—Evidence from a meta-analytic review. *Perspectives on Psychological Science, 11*(4), 512–534. https://doi.org/10.1177/1745691616635612

Miranda, M. C., Borges, M., & Rocca, C. C. A. (2018). Avaliação neuropsicológica infantil. In L. F. Malloy-Diniz, D. Fuentes, P. Mattos, & N. Abreu (Eds.), *Avaliação Neuropsicológica* (2a ed., pp. 206–217). Artmed.

Nery-Barbora, M., & Barbosa, D. M. (2017). Reabilitação da memória. In L. Malloy-Diniz, P. Mattos, N. Abreu, & D. Fuentes (Eds.), *Neuropsicologia aplicações clinicas* (pp. 272–290). Artmed.

Oliveira, J. C. (2014). O uso da CIF na avaliação neuropsicológica de uma criança com traumatismo cranioencefálico (TCE) (Trabalho de Conclusão de Curso, Universidade Federal do Rio Grande do Sul).

Otero, T., Barker, L., & Naglieri, J. A. (2014). Executive function treatment and intervention in schools. *Applied Neuropsychology: Child, 3*(3), 205–214. https://doi.org/10.1080/21622965.2014.897903

Palisano, R. J. (2006). A collaborative model of service delivery for children with movement disorders: A framework for evidence-based decision making. *Physical Therapy, 86*, 1295–1305.

Piccolo, L. R., Sbicigo, J. B., Grassi-Oliveira, R., & Salles, J. F. (2014). Do socioeconomic status and stress reactivity really impact neurocognitive performance? *Psychology & Neuroscience, 7*, 567–575. https://doi.org/10.3922/j.psns.2014.4.16

Pontes, L. M. M., & Hubner, M. M. C. (2008). A reabilitação neuropsicológica sob a ótica da psicologia comportamental. *Revista de Psiquiatria Clínica, 35*(1), 6–12. https://doi.org/10.1590/S0101-60832008000100002

Poser, U. (1996). Historical review of neuropsychological rehabilitation in Germany. *Neuropsychological Rehabilitation, 6*(4), 257–278.

Prigatano, G. P. (1986). The patient competency rating scale. In G. P. Prigatano (Ed.), *Neuropsychological rehabilitation after brain injury*. Johns Hopkins University Press.

Rajeswaran, J., Bennett, C. N., & Shereena, E. A. (2013). Neuropsychological rehabilitation: Need and scope. In J. Rajeswaran (Ed.), *Neuropsychological rehabilitation principles and applications* (pp. 1–10). Elsevier Science.

Rysdyk, E., Pureza, J. R., Gonçalves, H., Cardoso, C. O., & Fonseca, R. P. (2016). Programa PENcE: do Contexto Escolar ao Contexto Clínico. In C. O. Cardoso & R. P. Fonseca (Eds.), *Programa de Estimulação Neuropsicológica da Cognição em Escolares: ênfase nas Funções Executivas* (pp. 141–173). BookToy.

Sant'Anna, B. A., & Mello, C. B. (2017). Relato de caso—Reabilitação holística em pacientes pediátricos com lesão cerebral. In D. R. Fontoura, L. Tisser, O. Bueno, S. Bolognani, & T. Frison (Eds.), *Teoria e prática na reabilitação neuropsicológica* (pp. 69–80). Vetor.

Santos, F. H. (2005). Reabilitação neuropsicológica pediátrica. *Psicologia ciência e profissão, 25*(3), 450–461.

Santos, R. M., Toffoli, M. B., Cardoso, A. P. B., Drumond, G. P., & Rosa, D. A. (2006). *Pedro na casa mal-assombrada: desenvolvendo habilidades auditivas*. CTS Informática.

Santos, R. M., Toffoli, M. B., & Costa, A. C. (2008). *Pedro no parque de diversões: desenvolvendo consciência fonológica*. CTS Informática.

Santos, R. M., Prando, M. L., Frison, T. B., & Casarin, F. S. (2012). *Pedro no acampamento: habilidades neurocognitivas*. CTS Informática.

Scherf, K. S., Sweeney, J. A., & Luna, N. (2006). Brain basis of developmental change in visuospatial working memory. *Journal of Cognitive Neuroscience, 18*, 1045–1058.

Taylor, H. G., Yeates, K. O., Wade, S. L., Drotar, D., Stancin, T., & Minich, N. (2002). A prospective study of short-and long-term outcomes after traumatic brain injury in children: Behavior and achievement. *Neuropsychology, 16*(1), 15.

Thomson, J., Kerns, K., Seidenstrang, L., Sohlberg, M. M., & Mateer, C. A. (2005). *Pay attention! A children's attention process training program*. Lash.

Thorell, L. B., Lindqvist, S., Bergman Nutley, S., Bohlin, G., & Klingberg, T. (2009). Training and transfer effects of executive functions in preschool children. *Developmental Science, 12*(1), 106–113. https://doi.org/10.1111/j.1467-7687.2008.00745.x

Wada, J. A. (2009). Is functional hemispheric lateralization guided by structural cerebral asymmetry? *Canadian Journal of Neurological Sciences, 36*(Suppl2), S25–S31.

Wilson, B. (1989). Models of cognitive rehabilitation. In R. L. Wood & P. Eames (Eds.), *Models of brain injury rehabilitation*. Chapman & Hall.

Wilson, B. A. (1997). Cognitive rehabilitation: How it is and how it might be. *Journal of the International Neuropsychological Society, 3*, 487–496.

Wilson, B. A. (2002). Management and remediation of memory problems in brain-injured adults. In A. D. Baddeley, M. D. Kopelman, & B. A. Wilson (Eds.), *The handbook of memory disorders* (2nd ed., pp. 655–682). Wiley.
Wilson, B. A. (2008). Neuropsychological rehabilitation. *Annual Review Clinical Psychology, 4*, 141–162. https://doi.org/10.1146/annurev.clinpsy.4.022007.141212
Wilson, B. A., Gracey, F., Evans, J. J., & Bateman, A. (2009). *Neuropsychological rehabilitation: Theory, models, therapy and outcome*. Cambridge University Press.
Wilson, B., Winegardner, J., Van Heugten, C. M., & Ownsworth, T. (2017). *Neuropsychological rehabilitation: The international handbook*. Routledge.
World Health Organization—WHO. (2001). *International classification of functioning, disability and health: ICF*. World Health Organization.
Yeates, K. O., Taylor, H. G., Walz, N. C., Stancin, T., & Wade, S. L. (2010). The family environment as a moderator of psychosocial outcomes following traumatic brain injury in young children. *Neuropsychology, 24*(3), 345. https://doi.org/10.1037/a0018387

Chapter 3
Stimulation of Cognitive Functions in a School Context: Guidance for Teachers

Janice da Rosa Pureza

In recent years, significant attention has been given to the relationship between neuroscience, neuropsychology, and education. After all, how can the brain and education sciences contribute to the teaching and learning process? What does the educator need to know about cognition? How can the contributions of neuroscience and neuropsychology be applied in the classroom (Diamond, 2012; Guerra et al., 2004; Tokuhama-Espinosa, 2010)?

Since the 1990s, with the advancement of research and technologies that enabled a better understanding of the development, structure, and functioning of the brain, there has been a great interest in the circuits and brain regions involved in learning and its related cognitive processes, among these, attention, memory, language, and executive functions (Arruda, 2015; Rotta et al., 2016).

Attention is the cognitive function that allows the brain to process limited information in the individual's context. This skill allows the selection of stimuli to be processed, making it easier for the brain to make a judicious and sensible use of its cognitive resources. Attention is also responsible for monitoring the individual's interaction with their environment, whether through controlled or automatic processes, with a greater or lesser degree of awareness of the situation and using more or less attentional resources (Castro et al., 2010; Ocampo, 2009).

Among the various modalities of attention, concentrated attention stands out, which means maintaining attention on a certain stimulus, suppressing other concurrent information (listening attentively to the teacher's explanation in class instead of being interested in the children singing in the schoolyard), dividing attention, which is the ability to divide attentional focus between two simultaneous stimuli (riding a bicycle and talking on the phone at the same time); selective attention, which allows performing a task continuously in the presence of distracting stimuli (not hearing

J. R. Pureza (✉)
Conectare NeuroPsi, Porto Alegre, Brazil
e-mail: janicepureza@gmail.com

C. O. Cardoso, N. M. Dias (eds.), *Neuropsychological Interventions for Children - Volume 1*, https://doi.org/10.1007/978-3-031-53586-4_3

the phone ring when you are reading an interesting book); alternating attention, which allows performing tasks that require rapid changes in the response repertoire (sometimes the focus of attention is on the Portuguese activity, sometimes on the math task) (Castro et al., 2010; Ocampo, 2009).

Memory is the cognitive process responsible for the recording of information (*encoding*), for its maintenance for a specific period (*storage*) and for recalling this information later (*retrieval*) (Matlin, 2004; Smith & Kosslyn, 2013). It is an important cognitive process for learning, as it allows the acquisition and conservation of information and contents worked on in class. Among the various modalities, memory processes can be classified according to duration—long-term memory (information is stored for a long period of time) and short-term memory (storage of information for a short period of time); and according to content—declarative memory (its content comes easily to consciousness, such as words with meanings, learned and lived experiences) and non-declarative memory (unconscious, automatic information, like driving, for example) (Matlin, 2004; Pureza et al., 2016; Smith & Kosslyn, 2013).

Language is the cognitive function responsible for communication (expressing emotions and thoughts, allowing interaction between individuals) and can be classified by phonetics and phonology (related to sounds), semantics (meanings), syntax (arrangement of words in sentences), morphology (smallest unit of the word) and pragmatics (use of language in various contexts) (Harley, 2001). Language shares resources with other cognitive processes, such as memory, attention, and executive functions (Gooch et al., 2016; Pureza et al., 2016).

In turn, executive functions are understood as cognitive processes that control and regulate behaviors directed towards specific ends, enabling the individual's adaptation and performance in their environment. For this, they rely on the participation of various cognitive components such as cognitive flexibility, self-monitoring, organization, planning, initiation and inhibition of thoughts and behaviors, attention, and working memory, among others (Almy & Zelazo, 2015; Chan et al., 2008; Kerr & Zelazo, 2004; Muller et al., 2008).

In addition to the mentioned characteristics, executive functions are associated with the abilities of logical reasoning, abstraction, and problem-solving (fluid intelligence), enabling the child to critically analyze various situations and contexts and seek new alternatives for resolving impasses that may arise. Another important aspect to be considered is the relationship between the development of executive skills and the ability for self-regulation in childhood, allowing the child to regulate and manage their emotions and behaviors, adapt to environmental demands, and favor the process of social interaction (Diamond, 2013).

Diamond (2013) emphasizes the importance of inhibitory control, working memory, and cognitive flexibility among the components of executive functions. Inhibitory control is the ability to inhibit behaviors, emotions, and distracting thoughts that are out of context. It involves attention control (attentional inhibition), which is the ability to inhibit attention to irrelevant stimuli, like a child who stops paying attention to other conversations to listen to the teacher. It also includes interference control (cognitive inhibition), that is, the child's ability to resist distracting thoughts when they have to perform a task and also includes self-control, which is the child's ability to control their actions and emotions (Diamond, 2013).

Working memory is responsible for coordinating multiple information for the performance of activities, as it allows one to keep in mind information that can be manipulated (Baddeley et al., 2011; Diamond, 2013). For example, to solve a mathematical operation, the child needs to keep in mind the information (numbers and operations) to be able to do the calculations (manipulation and mental reorganization of information).

Cognitive flexibility is related to the change of strategies and direction of actions or thoughts to solve specific demands. It is the child's ability to shift the focus of attention between different ideas, seeking to meet their objectives in a more effective way (Lezak et al., 2012; Diamond, 2013).

In the school context, executive functions ensure that children can organize and plan in the face of multiple classroom demands, can seek alternative solutions to solve tasks in situations of impasse or greater complexity, can handle multiple information in the performance of an activity (text interpretation or mathematical operations), as well as, resist distracting stimuli to listen to the teacher's explanation (conversations, noises in the classroom). Among the executive processes, the components of working memory, inhibitory control (inhibition), and cognitive flexibility are considered fundamental for the organization, coordination, and performance of academic activities (Cardoso & Fonseca, 2016; Diamond, 2013; Dias & Seabra, 2013; Meltzer, 2010).

Studies show that a better understanding of neurocognitive/emotional development during childhood can be very useful for educators in the teaching-learning process, as it provides the teacher with new possibilities of action in front of their students, such as stimulating the capacity for autonomy and self-regulation and enhancing cognitive and metacognitive processes essential for the academic development of children (Bierman et al., 2008; Consenza & Guerra, 2011; Dias & Seabra, 2016; Jones et al., 2010; Meltzer & Basho, 2010; Pureza & Fonseca, 2016; Tokuhama-Espinosa, 2010).

Consequently, investment in approaches aimed at enhancing cognitive and emotional skills is increasingly being implemented in the school context (Bierman et al., 2008; Bodrova & Leong, 2007; Diamond, 2012; Cardoso & Fonseca, 2016; Carvalho & Abreu, 2023; Dias & Seabra, 2013; Jones et al., 2010; Meltzer & Basho, 2010; Pureza & Fonseca, 2016; Rosário et al., 2007). This chapter aims to present some reflections on how neuropsychology can contribute more effectively to teaching practice and children's academic performance. Why and how to stimulate cognitive skills in the classroom? It also intends to present some suggestions for stimulating these skills in a school context.

Why and How to Enhance Cognitive Skills in the School Context?

Is it possible to learn better? How to favor the learning process and ensure that children can meet their goals as students? (Diamond, 2013; Meltzer, 2010; Tokuhama-Espinosa, 2010). For a better understanding of these demands, one should consider how brain development and interactions with the environment can influence the evolution of learning.

From birth, the child's brain is composed of billions of neurons that are activated in the performance of motor or cognitive activities, transmitting information to each other through their axons and dendrites. These nerve cells' continuous and systematic stimulation enhances, reorganizes, and reinforces new information networks, favoring the learning process (Consenza & Guerra, 2011; Rotta et al., 2016; Vianin, 2013).

Consequently, the interactions and experiences lived by the child, whether in the family, school, or social context, contribute to the development and brain restructuring driven by cognitive activity (Consenza & Guerra, 2011; Rotta et al., 2016; Vianin, 2013). Factors such as age, education, type of school, socioeconomic conditions, and cultural conditions have an important relationship with neurocognitive development in childhood and can influence the evolution of cognitive and socio-emotional skills (Jacobsen et al., 2016; Rosseli & Ardila, 2003).

Regarding the school environment, various cognitive skills are required for learning, such as attention, memory, language, and especially executive functions, which are necessary to acquire reading, writing, and math skills, among other demands. Consider reading/writing as an example: This learning process requires the child to develop the cognitive and linguistic potential to focus on all elements of syllables/words, relating sounds to specific letters. Thus, in addition to linguistic skills, working memory is required for the maintenance and manipulation of verbal content, enabling the resolution of the task by the child (reading/writing) (Alloway et al., 2010; Cardoso et al., 2015; Silva & Capellini, 2013).

In reading and text comprehension activities, in addition to language and attention, working memory, cognitive flexibility, and inferential capacity allow the child to integrate the information contained in the text, as well as understand and reflect on the content read (Mata et al., 2007). Cognitive flexibility plays an important role in language development, contributing to the encoding and expression of mental representations (ideas and intentions). Language demands the participation of cognitive flexibility in the selection and encoding of new information in multiple contexts (Deák, 2003; Deák & Wiseheart, 2015).

Learning mathematics also involves attentional skills, memory, and executive functions, such as logical reasoning (establishing relationships between numbers and operations), working memory (retention of information and mental manipulation), abstraction, and cognitive flexibility in the resolution of operations and mathematical problems (Diamond, 2013; Freitas et al., 2010).

In general, executive processes are important for students to be able to handle assignments and projects and execute short- and long-term goals. These demands involve important skills for the student, such as organizational ability, planning, and self-monitoring in carrying out their activities and managing the time needed to execute them (Meltzer & Basho, 2010).

In addition, there are two skills that are related to executive functions. These are metacognitive and self-regulation skills. Children need to develop metacognitive skills, as it is necessary for the student to manage their cognitive processes and be able to reflect and evaluate their performance. Metacognition is the individual's ability to perceive, evaluate, and monitor their thoughts and behaviors, adapting to their proposed objectives (Corso et al., 2013; Dias & Seabra, 2013; Rosário et al., 2007). Self-regulation allows the child to perceive and recognize their emotions, feelings, thoughts, and physical sensations, and thus be able to inhibit automatic and irrelevant responses and adapt their actions according to environmental demand. Metacognition and self-regulation enable the child to effectively organize, monitor, and manage their cognition and behavior (Blair et al., 2005; Fuster et al., 2008).

The stimulation of cognitive, metacognitive, and self-regulation skills can and should be carried out in the classroom, contributing to a condition of greater autonomy and independence for the students (Meltzer & Basho, 2010). According to Meltzer (2010), some strategies adapted to the school curriculum can be used in class to enhance various cognitive skills and students' academic performance. Among these actions, the author emphasizes teaching cognitive strategies to encourage children to monitor, evaluate, and coordinate their performance in carrying out tasks. This teaching contributes to acquiring greater autonomy and developing self-regulation capacity (Meltzer, 2010).

It is important that cognitive strategies are conveyed with clear and objective language and are modeled through the performance of the teacher or through the child's own individual strategies (reflecting and evaluating results and performance). The teacher should monitor whether this learning is being systematically used to execute school tasks (Meltzer, 2010).

Regarding the stimulation of executive functions, Diamond (2012) emphasizes the importance of systematic repetition of strategies and the increase in the level of complexity of tasks as the child manages to achieve the established goals. Children need to be encouraged to always deal with new demands. Otherwise, the activity can become boring and unattractive. Direct and stimulating action by the teacher can improve executive, metacognitive, and self-regulation skills (Diamond, 2012; Meltzer, 2010).

Based on the studies presented, some programs aim to stimulate children's cognitive, emotional, and behavioral skills directed toward the school community. Among these approaches, the Promoting Alternative Thinking Strategies Program—PATHS Program (Greenberg et al., 1995; Riggs et al., 2006), the Head Star HEDI (Bierman et al., 2008), and the Chicago School Readiness Project—CSRP (Raver et al., 2011) stand out.

These programs aim to develop readiness for learning and prevent long-term disruptive behaviors. They are intended for preschool-aged children, stimulating executive functions and self-regulation as support for better school performance and socio-emotional adaptation of children (Biermann et al., 2008; Raver et al., 2011; Riggs et al., 2006). The teacher is guided to use specific classroom management strategies that aim to encourage self-monitoring skills, organization and planning, motivating children for the learning process (Biermann et al., 2008; Raver et al., 2011; Riggs et al., 2006).

Still referring to preschool-aged children, the programs *Tools of the Mind* (Bodrova & Leong, 2007) and *Sarrilhos do Amarelo* (Rosário et al., 2007) stand out. The *Tools of the Mind* program is based on the theories of Luria and Vygotsky about cognitive functioning and the importance of implementing structured strategies to develop executive and socio-emotional skills. It involves the teacher's mediating participation in implementing classroom strategies to stimulate executive skills, such as planning, self-monitoring, memory, attention, and socio-emotional skills (Bodrova & Leong, 2007).

The *Sarrilhos do Amarelo* program is intended for children aged 5–10 years, promoting self-regulation strategies and autonomy in the learning process through interactive activities focused on the Portuguese language and mathematics. Using a narrative approach, the program stimulates the ability to reflect and understand through stories, in addition to attentional processes, reasoning, and problem-solving skills (Rosário et al., 2007).

In the Brazilian context, as an example, the first program developed to stimulate self-regulation and executive functions for preschool-aged children was the Intervention Program in Self-Regulation and Executive Functions—PIAFEX (Dias & Seabra, 2013). This program has specific strategies to achieve its objectives, revisiting and enhancing approaches with theoretical support from other programs (Bodrova & Leong, 2007; Meltzer, 2010; Rosário et al., 2007). Among the strategies used, structured motor activities, specific techniques for enhancing executive skills, use of external mediators and private speech stand out, in addition to the important mediating, interactive, and modeling role of the teacher in implementing the activities (Dias & Seabra, 2013).

Another notable approach to stimulating executive functions and related cognitive processes is the Neuropsychological Stimulation Program of Cognition in Schoolchildren: Emphasis on Executive Functions—PENcE (Cardoso & Fonseca, 2016). PENcE has a set of strategies for stimulating executive functions in elementary school children. This program is executed by the teacher in the classroom and includes the systematic development of activities and strategies, such as: (a) fixed number of sessions; (b) time management in the execution of activities; (c) methodology in carrying out the activities (Cardoso & Fonseca, 2016).

The school community also has another program to stimulate executive skills in elementary school children. This is the Educator Training Program on Neuropsychology of Learning: Emphasis on Executive Functions and Attention—CENA (Pureza & Fonseca, 2016). CENA aims to educate and train educators to stimulate executive functions in the classroom. Through a training process, educators, with creativity and autonomy, can implement activities and strategies for stimulating executive functions in their students. CENA contributes to the educators' ability to apply knowledge from neuropsychology in their classroom practice, enhancing important cognitive functions for the learning process of their students (Pureza & Fonseca, 2016). Readers can refer to Chap. 9 of this work to deepen their reading about these and other stimulation programs of executive functions.

The range of programs presented highlights the importance of implementing early-preventive approaches, aiming to boost cognitive and socio-emotional skills in children in the school context. These preventive actions can prevent, minimize, or assist in detecting risk factors for development and the learning process in childhood. In addition, cognitive processes, such as executive functions, are considered general indicators of health, quality of life, academic and professional success, as well as contributing to the enhancement of socio-emotional skills (Diamond, 2012, 2013; Center on the Developing Child at Harvard University, 2011).

Suggestions to Enhance Cognitive Skills in the Classroom

Research shows that the adoption of specific arrangements can contribute to the development of cognitive, metacognitive, and self-regulation skills in the classroom (Biermann et al., 2008; Dias & Seabra, 2016; Meltzer, 2010; Riggs et al., 2006). In addition to the aspects emphasized in the previous section, such as some strategies adapted to the curriculum and the implementation of specific programs, certain actions can be carried out in the school space, with activities and resources available and experienced in the children's daily lives. Among these actions, the following stand out:

Physical Activities

Studies suggest that, regardless of age, systematic physical activity contributes to better executive performance (Diamond, 2012). In general, aerobic exercises are related to increased processing speed, cognitive flexibility, and greater ability in problem-solving strategies. Martial arts activities boost cognitive and emotional processes and stimulate adaptation to social rules (Center on the Developing Child at Harvard University, 2011; Diamond, 2012, 2015). The practice of physical activities, especially team sports, such as volleyball, soccer, and basketball, assist executive and self-regulation skills, contributing to socio-emotional skills and adaptation to the rules of each sport, stimulating self-monitoring and exercising decision-making by children (Center on the Developing Child at Harvard University, 2011; Diamond, 2012, 2015). One of the advantages of this type of activity is that it is part of the school curriculum through physical education and is practiced at various recreation times.

Activities with Music, Singing, and Dancing

In music classes, learning to sing or play a musical instrument is an interesting strategy to stimulate executive skills, self-monitoring, selective attention, and language. In addition to these skills, there is a demand for working memory, as the child needs to keep essential information from the music in their mind (lyrics, sequences of melodies). Musical activities require children to follow rhythmic patterns, particularly when the activity involves improvisation processes (for example, clapping or playing a specific instrument at certain parts of the music), requiring greater participation from working memory, attention, cognitive flexibility, and inhibitory control (Center on the Developing Child at Harvard University, 2011).

The modalities of singing groups for children require a joint performance of working memory, self-monitoring, and selective attention. Moreover, singing activities are fun challenges, and as children improve their musical skills, the level of challenges presented can increase (Center on the Developing Child at Harvard University, 2011).

Meditation

Meditation exercises are easy-to-apply activities in the school context and stimulate executive and self-regulation skills. Among the meditation modalities, yoga seems to enhance organization and planning skills. The modality of *mindfulness* has been related to better executive control and attentional skills (Diamond, 2012; Gothe et al., 2013). Studies suggest that the systematic practice of meditation exercises can improve academic performance and better prepare students to face future challenges (Diamond, 2012). Readers interested in this topic can consult Chap. 10 of Book 2 of Neuropsychological Interventions for Children, which will address mindfulness techniques.

Narrative Activities

Storytelling, retelling, and story creation activities demand various cognitive skills, such as selective and concentrated attention, episodic and semantic memory, and linguistic skills (verbal fluency, understanding and verbal expression, and synthesis ability). In addition to these processes, working memory is recruited (the child needs to keep in mind the main information of the story for retelling or creating a story), cognitive flexibility (to envision new possibilities of alternatives for resolving the story), and creativity for creating characters and situations (Cantiere et al., 2012; Pureza & Fonseca, 2016). This type of activity is easily applicable and is usually carried out in a school context. The systematic implementation of narrative activities, increasing the level of complexity as children meet the presented demands, can enhance cognitive processes important for learning.

Playful Activities

Card Games and Board Games

Games are interesting, playful activities for the enhancement of cognitive skills. In various forms, card games require executive skills, such as cognitive flexibility, for example, when the child needs to match cards by alternating criteria, such as suit, color, or number—game *Can Can*. Some card games demand quick responses from children, sometimes motor ones, stimulating attention, inhibitory control, and processing speed to meet the game's objectives—for example, games *Slap, Steal Pile* (Center on the Developing Child at Harvard University, 2011).

Board games, when they involve some type of strategy, require the child to plan and keep a goal in mind for the necessary steps in the moves, adjusting their strategies according to the moves of the opposing children—games *Checkers, Chinese Checkers, Chess, Ludo*. To elaborate the necessary strategies, the child needs the joint participation of working memory processes, inhibitory control, and flexibility to plan and execute their plans to win the games. This type of activity can be carried out in the classroom, contextualizing with some worked content or in moments of recreation (Center on the Developing Child at Harvard University, 2011).

Musical Games

Games with music usually involve motor activities and require children to be capable of self-control and quick actions. For example, there are musical chairs where the child must look for a chair and sit immediately when the music is interrupted. This type of game demands inhibitory and attentional control and orientation of their actions according to the rules of the game (Center on the Developing Child at Harvard University, 2011; Pureza & Fonseca, 2016).

Strategy and Reflection Games

Various games require reflective skills, search for strategies and problem-solving ability, emphasizing *Puzzle* games, *Mazes*, and games of *Logical Reasoning*. This type of activity is interesting because children, to achieve their goals in the games, need concentrated attention and working memory to keep all the necessary information in mind and cognitive flexibility to seek new actions if their strategies are not effective (Center on the Developing Child at Harvard University, 2011; Pureza & Fonseca, 2016).

Guessing Games

Guessing games are popular among children and demand components of attention, episodic and semantic memory, working memory, and cognitive flexibility, as the child needs to keep in mind the previous answers while they reflect and evaluate the need to change their answers or not. Among these games, "A trip to the moon" stands out, in which the child must plan what they will take for a trip to the moon. However, there are criteria for this selection, and the children must discover what these criteria are based on the clues provided, for example, by the teacher (Center on the Developing Child at Harvard University, 2011; Pureza & Fonseca, 2016).

The interested reader can also consult Chap. 12 of Volume 2 of Neuropsychological Interventions for Children, which will address the use of games and play in stimulating skills in childhood.

School Tasks for Cognitive Skill Stimulation

Cognitive skills can be stimulated in curricular activities, especially reading, writing and mathematics tasks. For example, to solve mathematical problems, children can be encouraged to reflect on the necessary steps for problem-solving and plan their execution, evaluating later if the strategies used were effective. The teacher stimulates the students by acting as a model in the execution of tasks (Cardoso & Fonseca, 2016). This strategy increases children's ability to organize, plan, and concentrate attention and reasoning.

The reading task is another school curriculum activity that can be adapted to stimulate cognitive skills. For example, the teacher can read a text aloud and out of order. The children need to put the text in the correct order for it to make sense (Cardoso & Fonseca, 2016). This type of activity mainly stimulates concentrated attention, working memory, and verbal understanding.

Numerous resources and activities can be used to enhance cognitive skills in the classroom. Many of these resources are specific programs for this purpose. However, playful or formal activities are available for the teacher's use. Some were exemplified in this chapter. However, most of these strategies and games are already widely used in the classroom. The difference is that a greater knowledge about neurocognitive development in childhood and how this evolution is important for the learning process allows the teacher to reinterpret their practice, combining objectives and playful strategies with cognitive stimulation of their students (Pureza & Fonseca, 2016).

Final Considerations

According to various studies, the intersection between neurosciences, more specifically, neuropsychology and the field of education, is being increasingly explored to contribute to a better learning process in childhood (Diamond, 2012;

Tokuhama-Espinosa, 2010). The stimulation of cognitive skills, such as attention, memory, language, and executive functions, can favor, in addition to a better academic performance, a better quality of life and a successful professional outcome.

In this sense, some approaches, such as the use of strategies adapted to the curriculum and the implementation of specific and systematic programs for stimulation, for example, of cognitive functions, are alternatives to enhance these skills in students (Diamond, 2012; Dias & Seabra, 2013; Meltzer, 2010). In addition, the training of educators provides greater knowledge about neurocognition in childhood. It allows greater autonomy and creativity for the teacher to plan and use strategies to enhance skills in their students, considering that various resources are available and are already experienced in the daily lives of children (Pureza & Fonseca, 2016).

This context reinforces the importance of conducting studies to encourage actions and programs to stimulate cognitive functions in a school setting. These interventions, in addition to contributing to better learning, can assist in the prevention or minimization of possible difficulties and/or learning disorders, as well as socio-emotional problems (Biermann et al., 2008; Dias & Seabra, 2016; Meltzer, 2010; Riggs et al., 2006). Consequently, greater investment at the interface of neuroscience, neuropsychology, and education can contribute to the adoption of public policies that aim to achieve better academic performance for our children.

References

Alloway, T. P., Banner, G. E., & Smith, P. (2010). Working memory and cognitive styles in adolescents attainment. *British Journal of Education Psychology, 80*, 567–581. https://doi.org/10.1348/000709910X494566

Almy, B. K., & Zelazo, P. D. (2015). Reflection and executive function: Foundations for learning and healthy development. *Revista Argentina de Ciencias del Comportamento, 7*(1), 53–59.

Arruda, M. A. (2015). Intervenções no contexto escolar. In N. M. Dias & T. P. Mecca (Eds.), *Contribuições da psicologia e da neuropsicologia para intervenção no contexto educacional* (Vol. 1, pp. 41–51). Memnon.

Baddeley, A. D., Anderson, M. C., & Eysenck, M. W. (2011). *Memória*. Artmed.

Bierman, K. L., Nix, R. L., Greenberg, M., Blair, C., & Domitrovich, C. E. (2008). Executive functions and school readiness intervention: Impact, moderation, and mediation in the Head Start REDI program. *Development and Psychopathology, 20*(3), 821–843. https://doi.org/10.1017/S0954579408000394

Blair, C., Zelazo, P. D., & Greenberg, M. T. (2005). The measurements of executive functions in early childhood. *Developmental Neuropsychology, 28*(2), 561–571. https://doi.org/10.1207/s15326942dn28021

Bodrova, E., & Leong, D. J. (2007). *Tools of the mind: The Vygotskian approach to earlychildhood education* (2nd ed.). Pearson.

Cantiere, C. N., Ribeiro, F. A., Khoury, L. P., Seraceni, M. F. F., Macedo, L. F. R., & Carreiro, L. R. R. (2012). Treino cognitivo em crianças e adolescentes com sinais de desatenção e hiperatividade: proposta de protocolo de intervenção neuropsicológica nos domínios verbal e executivo. *Cadernos de Pós-Graduação em Distúrbios do Desenvolvimento, 12*(1), 97–107.

Cardoso, C. O., & Fonseca, R. P. (2016). *Programa de estimulação neuropsicológica da cognição em escolares: ênfase nas funções executivas*. Book Toy.

Cardoso, C. O., Pureza, J. R., Gonçalves, H. A., Jacobsen, G., Senger, J., Colling, A. P. C., & Fonseca, R. P. (2015). Intervenções no contexto escolar. In N. M. Dias & T. P. Mecca (Eds.), *Contribuições da neuropsicologia e da psicologia para intervenções no contexto escolar* (pp. 63–81). Memnon.

Carvalho, C. F., & Abreu, N. (2023). *Heróis da Mente: caderno do aluno* (1st ed.). Ampla.

Castro, N. R., Rueda, F. J. M., & Sisto, F. F. (2010). Evidências de validade para o teste de atenção alternada—TEALT. *Pesquisa em Psicologia, 4*(01), 40–49.

Center on the Developing Child at Harvard University. (2011). *Building the brain's "air traffic control" system: How early experiences shape the development of executive function.*

Chan, R., Shum, D., Toulopoulou, T., & Chen, E. Y. H. (2008). Assessment of executive functions: Review of instruments and identification of critical issues. *Archives of Clinical Neuropsycholoy, 23*(2), 201–216. https://doi.org/10.1016/j.acn.2007.08.010

Consenza, R. M., & Guerra, L. B. (2011). *Neurociência e educação: como o cérebro aprende*. Artmed.

Corso, H. V., Sperb, T. M., Jou, G. I., & Salles, J. F. (2013). Metacognição e Funções Executivas: Relações entre os Conceitos e Implicações para a Aprendizagem. *Psicologia: Teoria e Pesquisa, 29*(1), 21–29.

Deák, G. O. (2003). The development of cognitive flexibility and language abilities. *Advances in Child Development and Behavior, 31*, 271–327.

Deák, G. O., & Wiseheart, M. (2015). Cognitive flexibility in young children: General or task-specific capacity? *Journal of Experimental Child Psychology, 138*, 31–53. https://doi.org/10.1016/j.jecp.2015.04.003

Diamond, A. (2012). Activities and programs that improve children's executive functions. *Current Directions in Psychological Science, 21*(5), 335–341. https://doi.org/10.1177/0963721412453722

Diamond, A. (2013). Executive functions. *Annual Review of Psychology, 64*, 135–168. https://doi.org/10.1146/annurev-psych-113011-143750

Diamond, A. (2015). Effects of physical exercise on executive functions: Going beyond simply moving to moving with thought. *Annals of Sports Medicine and Research, 2*(1), 1011.

Dias, N. M., & Seabra, A. G. (2013). *Programa de Intervenção em Autorregulação e Funções Executivas—Piafex*. Menmon.

Dias, N. M., & Seabra, A. G. (2016). Intervention for executive functions development in early elementary school children: Effects on learning and behavior and follow-up maintenance. *Educational Psychology, 37*(4), 468–486. https://doi.org/10.1080/01443410.2016.1214686

Freitas, N. L., Ferreira, F. O., & Haase, V. G. (2010). Linguagem e matemática: estudo sobre relações entre habilidades cognitivas linguísticas e aritméticas. *Ciências e Cognição, 15*(3), 111–125.

Fuster, D., Scholar, M., & Tan, P. Z. (2008). The relation between executive functioning and emotion regulation in young children. *The Penn State McNair Journal, 15*, 35–53.

Gooch, D., Thompson, P., Nash, H. M., Snowling, M. J., & Hulme, C. (2016). The development of executive function and language skills in the early school years. *The Journal of Child Psychology and Psychiatry, 57*(2), 180–187. https://doi.org/10.1111/jcpp12458

Gothe, N., Pontifex, M. B., Hillman, C., & McAuley, E. (2013). The acute effects of yoga on executive function. *Journal of Physical Activity and Health, 10*, 488–495.

Greenberg, M. T., Kushé, C. A., Cook, T., & Quamma, J. P. (1995). Promoting emotional competence in school-age children: The effects of the PATHS curriculum. *Development and Psychopatology, 7*, 117–136.

Guerra, L. B., Pereira, H. P., & Lopes, M. Z. (2004). *Neuroeduca: inserção da neurobiologia na educação*. Anais do 7° Encontro de Extensão da Universidade Federal de Minas Gerais.

Harley, T. A. (2001). *The psychology of language: From data to theory* (2nd ed.). Taylor & Francis.

Jacobsen, G. M., Prando, M. L., Moraes, A. L., Pureza, J. R., Gonçalves, H. A., & Siqueira, L. S. (2016). Effects of age and school type on unconstrained, phonemic and semantic verbal fluency in children. *Applied Neurpsychology Child, 0*, 1–14. https://doi.org/10.1080/21622965.2015.1072535

Jones, S. M., Zhai, F., & Raver, C. C. (2010). *Long-term impacts of the Chicago school readiness project on children's behavior in kindergarten school quality*. In Conference abstract template, society for research on educational effectiveness. www.sree.org
Kerr, A., & Zelazo, P. D. (2004). Development of "hot" executive function: The children's gambling task. *Brain and Cognition, 55*, 148–157.
Lezak, M. D., Howieson, D. B., Bigler, E. D., & Tranel, D. (2012). *Neuropsychological assessment* (5th ed., p. 1161). Oxford University Press.
Mata, F. G., Silva, J. B. L., & Haase, V. G. (2007). Narrativas: abordagens cognitivas e neuropsicológicas da análise da produção e compreensão. *Mosaico: Estudos em Psicologia, 1*(1), 51–59.
Matlin, M. W. (2004). *Psicologia cognitiva*. LTC.
Meltzer, L. (2010). *Promoting executive functions in the classroom*. Guilford.
Meltzer, L., & Basho, S. (2010). Creating a classroom wide executive function culture that fosters strategy use, motivation, and resilience. In L. Meltzer (Ed.), *Promoting executive function in the classroom* (pp. 28–54). Guilford.
Muller, U., Zelazo, P. D., Lurye, L. E., & Liebermann, D. P. (2008). The effect of labeling on preschool children's performance in the dimensional change card sort. *Cognitive Development, 23*(3), 395–408. https://doi.org/10.1016/j.cogdev.2008.06.001
Ocampo, L. P. L. (2009). La atención: un processo psicológico básico. *Revista de la Facultad de Psicología Universidad Cooperativa de Colombia, 5*(8), 91–100.
Pureza, J. R., & Fonseca, R. P. (2016). *CENA—Programa de capacitação de educadores sobre neuropsicologia da aprendizagem com ênfase em funções executivas e atenção*. Book Toy.
Pureza, J. R., Gonçalves, H. A., Pereira, N., & Fonseca, R. P. (2016). Estrutura e dinâmica do CENA. In J. R. Pureza & R. P. Fonseca (Eds.), *CENA—Programa de capacitação de educadores sobre neuropsicologia da aprendizagem com ênfase em funções executivas e atenção* (pp. 42–73). Book Toy.
Raver, C., Jones, S. M., Li-Grining, C., Zhai, F., & Pressler, E. (2011). CSRP's impact on low-income preschoolers' preacademic skills: Self-regulation as a mediating mechanism. *Child Devopment, 82*(1), 362–378. https://doi.org/10.1111/j.1467-8624.2010.01561.x
Riggs, N., Greenber, M. T., Kushé, C. A., & Pentz, M. A. (2006). The meditational role of neurocognition in the behavioral outcomes of a social-emotional prevention program in elementary school students: Effects of the PATHS curriculum. *Prevention Science, 7*(1), 91–102. https://doi.org/10.1007/s11121-005-0022-1
Rosário, P., Núñes, J. C., & González-Pienda, J. (2007). *Auto-regulação em crianças sub-10: Projecto sarilhos do amarelo*. Porto Editora.
Rosselli, M., & Ardila, A. (2003). The impact of culture and education on non-verbal neuropsychological measurements: A critical review. *Brian and Cognition, 52*, 326.
Rotta, N. T., Ohlweiler, L., & Riesgo, R. S. (2016). *Transtornos da aprendizagem: abordagem neurobiológica e multidisciplinar* (2nd ed.). Artmed.
Silva, C., & Capellini, S. A. (2013). Desempenho de escolares com e sem transtorno de aprendizagem em leitura, escrita, consciência fonológica, velocidade de processamento e memória de trabalho fonológica. *Revista de Psicopedagogia, 30*(91), 3–11.
Smith, E. E., & Kosslyn, S. M. (2013). *Cognitive psychology: Pearson New International Edition: Mind and brain*. Pearson Higher Education.
Tokuhama-Espinosa, T. (2010). *Mind, brain, and education science: The new brain-based learning* (1st ed.). W.W. Norton.
Vianin, P. (2013). *Estratégias de ajuda a alunos com dificuldades de aprendizagem*. Penso.

Chapter 4
Guidance to Parents and Psychoeducation: An Example from the Approach of Executive Functions

Marco Antônio Arruda

Tell me and I will forget
Show me and I may remember
Involve me and I will understand

Native American Proverb

The interface between Neuroscience and Education was officially marked by the foundation of the *International Mind, Brain, and Education Society* in 2006, a true milestone in the establishment of new paradigms in the field of Education based on the significant advancement of scientific knowledge about the brain and child development that occurred from 1990, the so-called decade of the brain. From then on, the broad interface of contact between Neuroscience and Education resulted in increasing research and advances that today allow the educational process, whether at home or in school, to be based on scientific evidence, leaving behind the "guesswork" of the past.

The Neuroscience of Education can be defined as a new branch of Neuroscience that studies education and the brain; this is understood as a social organ that can be modified by educational practice. Therefore, the brain is understood as a plastic organ at the mercy of positive (functional) and negative (dysfunctional) stimuli, being able to respond with the development of skills or difficulties in various areas of psychosocial and cognitive functioning.

The training of twenty-first-century parents and teachers in these knowledge and practices is of fundamental importance, as through educational interventions they can both stimulate skills and rehabilitate difficulties that the child may present.

We can divide this process into two stages, the first referring to identifying the skills and difficulties of each child within the whole diversity of child development;

M. A. Arruda (✉)
Glia Institute, Ribeirão Preto, Brazil
e-mail: arruda@institutoglia.com.br

C. O. Cardoso, N. M. Dias (eds.), *Neuropsychological Interventions for Children - Volume 1*, https://doi.org/10.1007/978-3-031-53586-4_4

the second related to the application of effective interventions in the stimulation and/or rehabilitation of fundamental competencies for human development.

But, After All, What Competencies Are We Talking About?

The literature is rich in evidence about the importance of executive functions (EF), in the first order, as a prerequisite for the development of more sophisticated skills such as problem-solving, delay of rewards and resilience, among others, which consequently will define more complex outcomes regarding mental health, behavior and learning. The early identification of children with EF difficulties allows early interventions that reduce the risk of them developing mental disorders and/or learning difficulties (Blair & Diamond, 2008; Diamond et al., 2007). By stimulating skills and rehabilitating difficulties, these interventions allow the attention of every child or teenager in their uniqueness, causing a great impact on the development of emotional regulation skills, behavioral control, and learning (Dias & Seabra, 2013).

The Importance of Teaching EF to Parents

Guiding parents and teachers on what EF are, how to identify them in the child's daily life at home and at school, and how, let's say here, to "educate them" is an essential task for the success of therapeutic interventions. In light of current evidence, it is impossible to separate the child's executive functioning from that of their family and social group; the high interactivity and influence exerted among these actors will determine not only performance but also the outcomes and therapeutic success of interventions. In a population study with a final sample of 3496 children aged 5–12 in the city of São Sebastião do Paraíso (MG), using functional scales of EF assessment, we found that children of parents who considered their home disorganized had a five times higher risk (Odds Ratio = 4.6; Confidence Interval 95% = 2.9–0.4) of EF problems compared to children whose parents considered their home well organized.

Scientific evidence proves that EF determines a series of extremely important outcomes in life. EF can be educated from an early age to prevent future deficits, rehabilitated in children who present them as deficient, and even enhanced in those whose performance is only average. To illustrate how we approach parents in a multidimensional EF intervention program we developed (Arruda et al., 2015), the introductory text is presented in Table 4.1.

In the aforementioned intervention program, called the Glia Method, we use the following paradigm that comprises 11 EF: goal setting, planning, organizing, initiating, focusing, persevering, monitoring, flexing, inhibiting, regulating, and operationalizing. In brochures specifically directed at parents and teachers, each of these EF is described through behaviors exhibited by the child in their daily life at home

Table 4.1 Introductory text of an EF intervention program

What are executive functions?
Imagine the multitude of experiences we live throughout life. From the comfort of the womb, through the birth canal, the first steps and words, to the first fall from a bicycle! Each experience we have is accumulated, combined with previous experiences, enabling new learning. This process gradually perfects itself and guides us through new experiences. We call executive functions the set of mental skills that regulate our behavior and thinking based on past experiences to perform actions in the present or achieve future goals. We extensively use these functions in our daily lives, whether to change clothes or to solve complex problems.
These highly sophisticated functions are processed on a carpet of cells that covers the front part of the brain, an area called the prefrontal cortex, but also involve the activation of several other brain circuits in sync.
Executive functions (EF) develop from birth until early adulthood and allow individuals to perform voluntary actions with autonomy and organization to achieve specific goals, hence their fundamental importance for behavior and school performance. We can compare EF to a soccer team with 11 players each with their distinct skills: Goal setting, planning, organizing, initiating, focusing, persevering, monitoring, flexing, inhibiting, regulating, and operationalizing. All these "players" work together, and when well-coordinated, they make wonderful plays and goals!

Taken from Arruda et al. (2015)

and at school. A story is also presented that contrasts the routine behaviors of a child with excellent executive functioning and another with difficulties in order to make the information more concrete for educators. Along with this material, Two 30-min videos are provided to parents, one about what EF are and another about how to educate them in their child's daily life (Arruda et al., 2015). The Glia Method also offers parents, teachers, and therapists a functional assessment of the child's EF and metacognitive skills through the completion of *online* questionnaires validated in the Brazilian child population; this is the instrument called AFFE (Functional Assessment of Executive Functions®) in its versions for parents and teachers (Arruda et al., 2022), and the AFMME (Functional Assessment of Metacognition and School Motivation®) in its version for completion by the literate child (Arruda & Arruda, 2018). Other instruments with a similar proposal are available internationally (Barkley, 2012; Gioia et al., 2000a, b; Naglieri & Goldstein, 2013). This naturalistic path of EF assessment has been gaining increasing space among specialists and researchers in the field (Barkley, 2012; Isquith et al., 2013).

The Importance of Parents Teaching EF to Their Children

Parents and teachers are in a privileged position to observe how diverse child development is in relation to EF. Some children are already "born ready," and their skills manifest daily as they develop and perform increasingly complex tasks. Others, from an early age, show difficulties in regulating their emotions, inhibiting behaviors, and learning, and over time, they end up failing in more complex tasks, making their difficulties apparent. These children and adolescents have difficulties in self-monitoring; in perceiving "*what, when, how, and why*" they failed and often end up mistakenly blaming others. Therefore, it is essential that throughout the interventions, parents, teachers, and/or therapists point out "*what, when, how, and why*" instead of expecting the child to become efficient through simple observation or by "osmosis" (Dawson & Guare, 2014). The interested reader can also consult Chap. 9 of this work for more information on stimulating EF.

A Metaphor About Executive Dysfunctions

The systematic monitoring of the literature and field research, combined with clinical experience in child and adolescent neuropsychiatry, qualifies us to propose a model for a better understanding of the universe of executive dysfunctions. Using the computer metaphor, we would have in the brain the *hardware* (equipment) with its memory devices and information processing, input and output paths, and in the habits and behaviors of the individual, the various *software* (programs) that run on this complex equipment. Well, in daily clinical practice we attend to children and adolescents who suffer from executive dysfunctions due to pathological mechanisms of neurobiological causes such as Attention Deficit Hyperactivity Disorder (ADHD), Learning Disorders, Anxiety and Mood Disorders, among others.

In the metaphor used here, these cases reflect problems in the functioning of the *hardware* and specific assessments of EF through neuropsychological tests reveal the malfunctioning of various brain circuits. This is a multifactorial condition whose resolution depends on multiple interventions, rehabilitation, and often, the use of medication. On the other hand, a significant and growing number of children and adolescents with behavioral and/or learning problems are brought to care. However, they do not meet clinical criteria for diagnosing these disorders. These children and adolescents exhibit the same dysfunctional behaviors as the first ones, but their neuropsychological tests often do not reveal any cognitive abnormality, including EF. According to our metaphor, this group has problems with software, and not *hardware*, that is, programming problems and not equipment problems. The executive dysfunctions occur because of dysfunctional habits and behaviors that must be reprogrammed. A very common example is that of a teenager who in neuropsychological tests presents a normal performance of organization. However, his room is a total mess; he can't organize his activities throughout the day and always arrives late to his appointments.

Very often these children and teenagers lacked the appropriate stimulus through the educational process; unfortunately, they are delegated to third parties whose executive skills are not often prerequisites in hiring. Other times these children and teenagers were adequately stimulated but did not develop healthy executive habits for various reasons. A third group can also be identified when unfavorable educational conditions are combined with the neurobiological disorder. This is the group of patients in which we face the greatest challenge in the rehabilitation and treatment process because often the parents and other caregivers are also dysfunctional and, occasionally, also have mental disorders. Whatever the group, the dynamics proposed here can be of great utility as long as the therapist can involve the patient, their parents, caregivers, and teachers in the intervention process.

Start from External to Internal Control

The development of EF occurs through the gradual internalization of "*what, when, how, and why*." This process begins with modeling the child's behaviors from efficient external stimuli and supervision at the appropriate time of development. Thus, initially, the parents hold the child's hand when crossing the street. Later, they verbally guided them ("look both ways before crossing"), and then they supervised them in the target task, finally letting them do it safely and independently. The therapist should guide the parents about this process so that the intervention initiatives at home have the desired success.

Everyone Involved Needs to Accept Changes

Executive functioning involves numerous factors, from innate and neurobiological (neuropsychiatric disorders, substance use, continuous medication use, etc.) to educational, including environmental, socioeconomic, and cultural aspects. As much as possible and at the right time, the therapist needs to expand their knowledge about the child and their habitat; after all, what is the executive functioning of the family as a whole? Working for a child to start to organize better in a disorganized house is like wanting a child to have the habit of reading when their parents do not read.

For the success of interventions in EF, whether in the early stimulation of the child with normal executive performance or in the rehabilitation of children and teenagers with executive dysfunctions, parents need to be aware of the need to modify the environment, behaviors, tasks, and the way they interact with their children. The child or teenager needs to accept the idea of modifying their behaviors and, above all, their way of thinking for better development. In turn, the school and the teacher need to be flexible, open to new things, and trained for the appropriate care of child diversity.

The Therapist Providing Support, Supervision, and Encouragement to Parents

Parents and other educators often make mistakes when supporting a child, either by providing too much; or insufficiently, making the development of the desired skill impossible. The secret is to check how far the child can perform the desired task independently and then intervene, not doing the task for the child but providing physical or verbal support (depending on the nature of the task) and sufficient supervision until they achieve the expected goal. Both support and supervision should be gradually withdrawn, never abruptly (Dawson & Guare, 2014). On the other hand, maintaining support and supervision for a longer time than necessary can convey insecurity to the child, ruining the success of the intervention.

Incentives are rewards that can be as simple as compliments or words of support or as complex as a point system that rewards the child on a daily, weekly, or monthly frequency based on pre-established goals (Dawson & Guare, 2014). Depending on the skill in play, for many children, achieving the proposed goal is, in itself, reward enough, such as learning to climb stairs, ride a bike, or start a game on the computer. However, many of the skills we want the child to develop do not incorporate attractive, let alone immediate, rewards. In these cases, the incentives should be established keeping in mind the motivation aroused by the task, its degree of difficulty, as well as the reward expectations demonstrated by the child. Here, again, incentives should be gradually withdrawn as soon as the child or teenager performs the task effectively and efficiently. Keeping the incentive for longer than necessary can awaken the child's obligation of this "exchange" to perform tasks that should be internalized and executed almost automatically. Not giving enough incentive can compromise the success of the intervention and the child's or teenager's confidence in their ability to develop skills (Dawson & Guare, 2014).

Interventions with parents to consequently reach the children are also of a psychotherapeutic order and, as such, have the essential element for their success in the quality of relationships with all parties involved. Essential, but not sufficient. It is crucial that there is integration of interventions with the relationships being built. This will allow the interventions to strengthen the relationships and, reciprocally, the strength of the relationships make the interventions effective (Friedberg et al., 2009).

Excessive formality, exaggerated pressure, impatience, or inflexibility can undermine the quality of relationships, putting the success of the interventions at risk (Creed & Kendall, 2005). On the other hand, the therapist's curiosity, sensitivity, and creativity are qualities that enrich relationships, amplifying the possibilities of intervention success (Friedberg et al., 2009).

Emotional Alert

The impact of emotions on memory and learning has been widely documented in the literature for more than a decade (Damasio, 1994; LeDoux, 1996, 2008). Thus, parents should be advised that, as interventions are carried out with the child or teenager, making him/her as alert as possible from an emotional point of view, the greater the success to be expected from the intervention. When the therapist also manages to trigger and, with heightened sensitivity, process the deepest emotions of the patient and their parents, the interventions are ready to take off (Friedberg et al., 2009).

Psychoeducation

Psychoeducation is a treatment modality that integrates educational and psychotherapeutic interventions (Lukens & McFarlane, 2004). In contrast to psychosocial interventions, which are based on the traditional medical model of disease treatment, psychoeducation proposes a paradigm shift to a more holistic and competency-based approach, valuing health, collaboration, coping, and empowerment of the patient and their family (Dixon, 1999).

Psychoeducation focuses on the present and the patient's strengths, he/she and his/her family become essential collaborators for the success of mental disorder treatment or behavioral modification, with the premise that the more knowledge these actors have about the condition they intend to intervene in, the greater the efficacy of the intervention. The actors' training for this partnership occurs through the application of psychoeducational techniques that will, on one side, facilitate the understanding of often complex information and high emotional-affective content and, on the other, develop strategies for proactive use of this information (Lukens & McFarlane, 2004).

It is one of the most effective evidence-based interventions with a broad spectrum of applications, whether in clinical conditions that affect general and/or mental health or in other challenges that life imposes (Lukens & McFarlane, 2004). The importance of psychoeducation is also justified by the source of hope it represents to the patient and their parents who, most of the time, arrive at the therapist with their relationships worn out and without prospects for resolution of the problem (Goldfried & Davila, 2005).

Psychoeducation is an indispensable initial step for cognitive-behavioral intervention. For it to be effective, psychoeducation cannot have the vertical and traditional teaching model of classrooms where the teacher (therapist) speaks and the students (patient and their family) listen; on the contrary, it must be quite interactive and fun. For this we suggest a vast list of activities that can be applied by the therapist or the parents themselves under the therapist's guidance, with a psychoeducational purpose, using websites, books, videos, movies, games and electronic and non-electronic games. For the process to be active, the therapist must see the patient and their parents not as mere recipients of information but as active consumers of this new information (Friedberg et al., 2009).

Other special tips for the success of this process:

(a) The materials or activities must contain relevant, useful information, culturally appropriate and engaging, compatible with the child's age and development.
(b) Instead of technical jargon, use stories, anecdotes and metaphors to facilitate the understanding and internalization of the concepts intended to be instilled.
(c) The therapist should always have in mind the conceptualization of the case, that is, the executive dysfunctions and psychological and social difficulties identified throughout the evaluation process.

It is interesting that the therapist assigns homework to the child and their parents already in this phase of psychoeducation, instilling the multipoint sense of the intervention, the transposition of what is discussed in the *therapeutic setting* (safe space where the client is welcomed in their way of being) to the necessary modifications in daily life. These tasks can be reading, internet research, games, movies, etc.; whenever possible, they should promote debate between the parties, whether between the child or adolescents and their parents or between them and the therapist.

Education About Child Development

How to perceive that certain behaviors or habits are appropriate for a certain stage of a child's development? How to understand the reasons for this inadequacy? How to convince yourself that something needs to be done? How to be trained to intervene in this process of modification? These and other questions have their answer in psychoeducation, more specifically in the education of parents and caregivers about the child's cognitive, affective, and behavioral development.

In this training process, the therapist should prioritize the paradigm of functionality, helping parents see their children holistically and from the perspective of what is functional or dysfunctional for them. A child can have extremely agitated behavior without suffering negative consequences for their social or academic functioning. On the other hand, a child without behavioral changes but with severe executive dysfunctions causing school and social failure needs to be promptly identified and receive interventions. Therefore, it is not about "labeling" a child as normal or abnormal; this reductionism does not translate the complexity of the child development process, creating barriers to effective interventions. Several sources of information are provided later in this chapter for the training of parents about child development.

Affective Education

Affective education is another key element in psychoeducation and teaches the child or adolescent and their parents to identify, understand and monitor the diversity of their emotions, the initial step for their adequate expression and emotional regulation (Friedberg et al., 2009).

Scientific evidence points to the importance of identifying emotions in developing emotional regulation (Suveg et al., 2006). For this identification, it is essential that the child has developed throughout their childhood skills that together we call the theory of mind, which is the ability of the individual to attribute mental states (emotions, intentions, desires, thoughts, knowledge, etc.) to themselves and others, and understand that they can be distinct (Premack & Woodruff, 1978; Tomasello, 2018). Such skills are indispensable for the cognitive, social, and emotional development of the child and are compromised to varying degrees in mental disorders such as Autism Spectrum Disorder, ADHD, and anxiety disorders, among others.

The therapist should be alert to identify and rehabilitate dysfunctions in these skills for the intervention to be successful (the reader can refer to Chap. 10 of this work for more information on interventions in the theory of mind).

Affective education can be conducted through various resources like movies, books, and music, with sociocultural, religious, and developmental content appropriate for the patient in question. In fact, such resources can be invaluable, given the interaction, motivation, and emotional alertness they provide, both for children and adolescents as well as for adults. However, it is recommended that the therapist always obtain the parents' permission before intervening with this type of resource (Friedberg et al., 2009). Affective education aims to develop empathy in the child or adolescent, a fundamental tool for their psychosocial adjustment and self-regulation (also refer to Chap. 11 on stimulation of socio-emotional skills).

Education About the Cognitive-Behavioral Model

The psychotherapeutic interventions with the best evidence of efficacy in the rehabilitation of EF are cognitive-behavioral based (Cardoso et al., 2018; Otero et al., 2014; Riccio & Gomes, 2013; Wass, 2015). Cognitive-behavioral therapy (CBT) is based on two central principles: our cognitions have a controlling influence over our emotions and behavior, and the way we act or behave can profoundly affect our patterns of thought and our emotions (Wright et al., 2008).

The rationale is to offer the patient a way to identify, understand, and modify their behaviors and emotions from a better understanding of their cognition. Educating the child or adolescent and their parents about the cognitive model and its applications greatly facilitates the interventions proposed here, amplifying the chances of success, whether by modifying dysfunctional behaviors and emotions or rehabilitating or enhancing the EF.

The cognitive model establishes that psychological difficulties arise from the interaction of four integrated areas of functioning: emotional, neurobiological, behavioral, and cognitive (Wright et al., 2008). Each of them influences and is influenced by the others in a relationship of mutual interaction. The classic telephone metaphor helps us better understand how this model works (Friedberg & Wilt, 2010). When we hear the phone ring, we immediately wonder who is calling us, why, and how we will react. The school principal? A friend's mother? Perhaps that ex-friend? What feeling occurs to us for each person we think is calling us? Fear, worry, or anger could be some alternatives. But after all, what thoughts (cognition) are behind these feelings? Is there evidence that supports this interrelation? What kind of feelings, anguish, and thoughts would occur if the person who was finally calling was not any of those imagined, but a dear friend with whom we haven't spoken in a long time?

This metaphor illustrates well that in different situations, we react with different feelings and thoughts that end up interfering with our behavior and emotions. Using this metaphor, the therapist can suggest to the child and/or their parents to write the situation in four columns, the feelings and thoughts that occur to them, and the resulting behavior. This can be a good start for understanding the cognitive-behavioral model.

When instructing a child or adolescent about this model, the therapist should highlight the key points of this intervention (Friedberg et al., 2009):

1. The physical, emotional, cognitive, and behavioral spheres are deeply related in such a way that changes in one directly contribute to modifications in the others.
2. Making sense of the world is a natural human process.
3. Sometimes this interpretation process is inaccurate and dysfunctional.
4. When the conclusions are correct, we will solve the problems together.
5. When they are incorrect, we will work together for you to formulate them better.
6. Behavioral rehearsals and experiments ("adventures") will be developed to test your conclusions.

When instructing the parents of the child or adolescent about the essence of the interventions, the therapist can use another metaphor, that of the fan (Friedberg et al., 2009). The loyal fan follows and believes in their team; regardless of the results they achieve, whether in victories or defeats, he is always there to give his support. The fan recognizes that rarely is a team unbeatable or a perfect player. Despite moments of suffering, the loyal fan remains optimistic. The same way is or should be the parents! Like all human beings, children are always subject to error and loss of control, especially when they go through stages of development where their emotional regulation and behavioral inhibition skills are not yet fully operational. Parents, like fans, can never give up, lose hope, or despair about their children.

Information Sources in Psychoeducation

Below are some information sources that can be used during the psychoeducation process.

Websites

- *Child development:* Núcleo Ciência pela Infância (www.ncpi.org.br).
- Encyclopedia on early childhood development (www.enciclopedia-crianca.com).
- Maria C. S. Vidigal Foundation for Early Childhood (www.fmcsv.org.br).
- Absolute Priority—Alana Institute (www.prioridadeabsoluta.org.br).
- ABCD Institute—Everyone Learns Program (www.todosaprendem.com.br).
- Center on the Developing Child—Harvard University (www.developingchild.harvard.edu).
- Educational activities (www.atividadeseducativas.com.br).

Useful Electronic Games for EF

Various games can be used, such as:

- Silversphere (Objective, Plan, Organize, Focus, Persevere and Monitor).
- Digital Switch (Objective, Plan, Initiate, Focus, Monitor, Flex and Inhibit).
- Aengie Quest (Objective, Plan, Organize, Focus and Persevere).

- Gude Balls (Objective, Plan, Initiate, Focus, Persevere, Monitor, Flex, Inhibit and Operationalize).
- Block Drop (Objective, Plan, Focus, Monitor and Inhibit).

Some links to access electronic games:

www.superjogosinfantis.com.br/blog
www.clicljogos.com.br/jogos-infantis
www.ojogos.com.br/jogos/infantil
www.papajogos.com.br/jogos-infantis
www.kids.pplware.sapo.pt/kids/apps-to-help-children-with-learning-difficulties-part-i

In addition to online games, video games can also be used in the interventions. Among the various options, the Wii is one of the most recommended, given the simplicity of its interface, the wide variety of games it offers and, above all, the innovative interaction that allows the player to control their digital actions through body movements (the Chap. 9 of Book 2 on Neuropsychological Intervention for Children will specifically address the use of games and digital technologies in neuropsychological stimulation).

Non-electronic Games and Play

- "Jocket." EF in play: focus, inhibit and monitor
- "Colorful little elephant." EF in play: target, focus and flexibilize
- "Follow the leader." EF in play: target, focus, inhibit, persist (engage), flexibilize, and monitor
- "Nice to meet you." EF in play: target, plan, organize (thought and time), inhibit, monitor, regulate and operate
- "Treasure hunt." EF in play: all EF
- "Stop." EF in play: all EF

Among the games, examples that involve various EF can be mentioned: Ice Breaker (from 3 years old), Pick Up Sticks (from 4 years old), Trap (from 5 years old), Don't Fall (from 5 years old), Genius (from 5 years old), Peg Solitaire (from 5 years old), SUDOKU (from 6 years old), Guess Who (from 6 years old), Tangram (from 6 years old), UNO (from 7 years old), Chess (from 7 years old), Mastermind (from 8 years old), Clue (from 8 years old), WAR (from 10 years old) and Profile 5 (from 12 years old) among others (the Chap. 12 of Volume 2 on Neuropsychological Interventions for Children will address games and play in the process of neuropsychological stimulation).

Children's Books and EF That Can Be Worked On

- "Little Red Riding Hood": inhibit, regulate and monitor
- "Fantastic Fables" (Elenice Machado de Almeida): target, plan, organize, initiate, focus, persist, monitor, flexibilize, inhibit, regulate and operate
- "I did what I could" (Lucília J. de Almeida Prado): persist, monitor, focus and target

- “Hansel and Gretel”: inhibit, regulate, monitor, plan, organize, focus and persist
- “Look at the girl’s eye” (Ziraldo): inhibit, regulate, monitor and flexibilize
- “The Three Little Pigs”: target, plan, organize, focus, monitor and flexibilize
- “Mary Poppins” (P. L. Travers): inhibit, regulate, monitor, organize and initiate
- “At the bakery door” (Ivan Zigg and Marcello Araujo): inhibit, regulate and monitor
- “Not a Box” (Antoinette Portis): flexibilize
- “Nicolau had an idea” (Ruth Rocha): operationalize, monitor and flexibilize
- “Pinocchio” (Carlo Collodi): inhibit, regulate and monitor

Children’s and Young Adult Books and EF that Can Be Worked On

- “Alice in Wonderland” (Lewis Carroll): persist, goal setting, monitor, flexibilize, inhibit, regulate, and operationalize
- “Alice Through the Looking Glass” (Lewis Carroll): goal setting, organize, focus, persist, flexibilize, and operationalize
- “The Adventures of Tom Sawyer” (Mark Twain): goal setting, organize, plan, focus, persist, monitor, flexibilize, inhibit, regulate, and operationalize
- “The Adventures of Huckleberry Finn” (Mark Twain): plan, organize, focus, persist, monitor, inhibit and regulate
- “Animal Farm” (George Orwell): goal setting, plan, organize, initiate, focus, persist, monitor, and flexibilize
- “The Time Machine” (H.G. Wells): goal setting, organize, initiate, focus, persist, monitor, and flexibilize
- “The Little Prince” (Antoine de Saint-Exupéry): goal setting, focus, persist, monitor, flexibilize, and operationalize
- “The Mystery of the Green House” (Moacyr Scliar): goal setting, organize, plan, initiate, focus, persist, monitor, inhibit, and regulate
- “The Devil’s Beetle” (Lucia Machado de Almeida): goal setting, plan, organize, initiate, focus, persist, monitor, and operationalize
- “Did the criminals come for tea?” (Stella Carr): goal setting, plan, organize, focus, persist, and monitor

Videos

- “Changing Brains.” Produced by Professor Helen J. Neville, Director of the Brain Development Laboratory at the University of Oregon (USA) and one of the world’s leading authorities on development and neuroplasticity. https://bdl.uoregon.edu/changing-brains-2/changing-brains-overview/
- “Three fundamental concepts about development in early childhood.” (www.ncpi.org.br/products/videos/)
- “Building adult skills to improve child performance” (www.ncpi.org.br/products/videos/)
- “The first thousand days of children” (www.youtube.com/watch?v=90D56DzIz1Q).

References

Arruda, M. A., Arruda, R., & Anunciação, L. (2022). Psychometric properties and clinical utility of the executive function inventory for children and adolescents: a large multistage populational study including children with ADHD. Applied *Neuropsychology, Child, 11*(1), 1–17.

Arruda, M. A., & Arruda, R. (2018). *Functional evaluation of metacognition and school motivation in children and adolescents: Psychometric properties of a new instrument.* Developed Instrument.

Arruda, M. A., Pinheiro, C. Q., Barros, C., Mata, M. F., Rezende, G., & Arroyo, L. H. (2015). *Método Glia: Cartilha dos Pais e do Professor*. Ed. Instituto Glia.

Barkley, R. (2012). *The Barkley deficits in executive functions scale—Children and adolescents.* Guilford.

Blair, C., & Diamond, A. (2008). Biological processes in prevention and intervention: The promotion of self-regulation as a means of preventing school failure. *Development and Psychopathology, 20*(3), 899–911. https://doi.org/10.1017/S0954579408000436

Cardoso, C. O., Dias, N., Senger, J., Colling, A. P. C., Seabra, A. G., & Fonseca, R. P. (2018). Neuropsychological stimulation of executive functions in children with typical development: A systematic review. *Applied Neuropsychology: Child, 7*(1), 61–81. https://doi.org/10.1080/21622965.2016.1241950

Creed, T. A., & Kendall, P. C. (2005). Therapist alliance-building behavior within a cognitive-behavioral treatment for anxiety in youth. *Journal of Consulting and Clinical Psychology, 73*(3), 498–505. https://doi.org/10.1037/0022-006X.73.3.498

Damasio, A. (1994). *Descartes' error: Emotion, reason, and the human brain.* Putnam, 1994; revised Penguin edition, 2005, 1994.

Dawson, P., & Guare, R. (2014). In S. G. J. A. Naglieri (Ed.), *Handbook of executive functioning*. Springer.

Diamond, A., Barnett, W. S., Thomas, J., & Munro, S. (2007). Preschool program improves cognitive control. *Science, 318*(5855), 1387–1388. https://doi.org/10.1126/science.1151148

Dias, N. M., & Seabra, A. G. (2013). *Programa de intervenção em autorregulação e funções executivas: Piafex*. Memnon.

Dixon, L. (1999). Providing services to families of persons with schizophrenia: Present and future. *Journal of Mental Health Policy and Economics, 2*, 3–8.

Friedberg, R. D., & Wilt, L. H. (2010). Metaphors and stories in cognitive behavioral therapy with children. *Journal of Rational-Emotive & Cognitive-Behavior Therapy, 28*, 100–113.

Friedberg, D., McClure, J. M., & Garcia, J. H. (2009). *Cognitive therapy techniques for children and adolescents*. Guilford.

Gioia, G., Isquith, P. K., Guy, S. C., & Kenworthy, L. (2000a). *Behavior rating inventory of executive function—Professional manual*. PAR.

Gioia, G., Isquith, P. K., Guy, S. C., & Kenworthy, L. (2000b). Test review: Behavior rating inventory of executive function. *Child Neuropsychology, 6*, 235–238. https://doi.org/10.1076/chin.6.3.235.3152

Goldfried, M. R., & Davila, J. (2005). The role of relationship and technique in therapeutic change. *Psychotherapy: Theory, Research, and Practice, 42*, 421–430.

Isquith, P. K., Roth, R. M., & Gioia, G. (2013). Contribution of rating scales to the assessment of executive functions. *Applied Neuropsychology: Child, 2*(2), 125–132. https://doi.org/10.1080/21622965.2013.748389

LeDoux, J. (1996). *The emotional brain: The mysterious underpinnings of emotional life*. Simon & Schuster.

LeDoux, J. (2008). *The Jossey-Bass reader on the brain and learning*. Wiley.

Lukens, E. P., & McFarlane, W. R. (2004). Psychoeducation as evidence-based practice: Considerations for practice, research, and policy. *Brief Treatment and Crisis Intervention, 4*(3), 205–255.

Naglieri, J. A., & Goldstein, S. (2013). *Comprehensive executive function index*. Multi-Health Systems.

Otero, T. M., Barker, L. A., & Naglieri, J. A. (2014). Executive function treatment and intervention in schools. *Applied Neuropsychology: Child, 3*(3), 205–214. https://doi.org/10.1080/21622965.2014.897903

Premack, D. G., & Woodruff, G. (1978). Does the chimpanzee have a theory of mind? *Behavioral and Brain Sciences, 1*, 515–526.

Riccio, C. A., & Gomes, H. (2013). Interventions for executive function deficits in children and adolescents. *Applied Neuropsychology: Child, 2*(2), 133–140. https://doi.org/10.1080/21622965.2013.748383

Suveg, C., Kendall, P. C., Comer, J. S., & Robin, J. (2006). Emotion-focused cognitive-behavior therapy for anxious youth: A multiple baseline evaluation. *Journal of Contemporary Psychotherapy, 36*, 77–86.

Tomasello, M. (2018). How children come to understand false beliefs: A shared intentionality account. *Proceedings of the National Academy of Sciences of the United States of America, 115*(34), 8491–8498. https://doi.org/10.1073/pnas.1804761115

Wass, S. V. (2015). Applying cognitive training to target executive functions during early development. *Child Neuropsychology, 21*(2), 150–166. https://doi.org/10.1080/09297049.2014.882888

Wright, J. H., Basco, M. R., & Thase, M. E. (2008). *Aprendendo a terapia cognitivo-comportamental: um guia ilustrado*. Artmed.

Chapter 5
How to Stimulate Cognitive, Emotional, and Behavioral Skills in the Clinical Context? General Guidelines to Therapists

Ariane Cristina Ramello de Carvalho

Developing and implementing a neuropsychological intervention can be a great challenge, as in addition to all the necessary theoretical knowledge, the therapist must build within themselves the necessary skills to be a good interventionist. Among these skills are planning, organization, cognitive flexibility, creativity, and a fundamental ingredient: theoretical and practical knowledge. These skills will significantly contribute to associating complaints, demands, and neuropsychological evaluation results to list goals and intervention strategies and their consequent systematization. In this way, the therapist will be able to be pragmatic, without losing sensitivity and flexibility, during the implementation of the intervention to not lose focus. Another challenge is knowing how to deal with the various demands arising from different types of clinical conditions or even complaints that do not necessarily establish a pathological condition but point to the need for better development of specific skills. Therefore, the objective of this chapter is to guide therapists in planning, goal selection, and use of strategies in the neuropsychological intervention process, as well as monitoring the results achieved.

Why Stimulate Skills in Children in the Clinical Context?

In general, neuropsychological stimulation or rehabilitation consists of using a series of techniques and strategies aimed at helping the individual to better cope with their cognitive deficits or even reduce them to have better efficiency in their academic activities or even daily life. It is an attempt to promote functional plasticity to reorganize the functionality of the person who presents some alteration or low performance in their cognitive skills (Abrisqueta-Gomez, 2012a; Ferreira, 2012).

A. C. R. de Carvalho (✉)
Universidade São Francisco, Campinas, Brazil
e-mail: ariane.ramello@gmail.com

C. O. Cardoso, N. M. Dias (eds.), *Neuropsychological Interventions for Children - Volume 1*, https://doi.org/10.1007/978-3-031-53586-4_5

The distinction between the terms neuropsychological rehabilitation and neuropsychological habilitation is highlighted here. When there is an alteration in cognitive processes due to a neurological or psychiatric condition due to any eventuality, the term neuropsychological rehabilitation is used (Wilson, 2017). On the other hand, when there is no neurological condition or event causing the loss of a skill or a set of skills, the intervention is framed within the scope of neuropsychological habilitation so that there is the development of skills that have not yet been acquired or do not perform well (Gindri et al., 2012). The interested reader can deepen their reading on this in Chap. 2 of this work.

With children and adolescents, it is very common to need an intervention that promotes habilitation to help the patient acquire and/or develop skills that assist in a more efficient performance in daily activities, according to the demands of the environment in which the child and adolescent live. In addition, currently, preventive interventions have gained notoriety for the fact that they are proving to be very effective in strengthening and improving cognitive, social, and emotional processes in children who present typical development (Cardoso et al., 2017; Gindri et al., 2012).

In this sense, Diamond (2015) emphasizes that despite human development being constructed by different aspects, it needs to be seen as a whole and not in a fragmented way. After all, cognitive, social, emotional, and physical components are intimately interrelated with mental health and academic performance, for example.

Given this, it is possible to perceive how important the clinical view on the demand of each patient is, as well as providing a therapeutic environment that is safe, organized, and capable of offering the child conditions to feel functionally active, healthy, and capable of facing challenges throughout their development (Abrisqueta-Gomez, 2012b; Frison et al., 2017).

That said, it is important to keep in mind that neuropsychological rehabilitation and/or stimulation is not a simple treatment or recovery but rather a process that promotes active changes in a person who has become incapable or who has begun to present difficulties in developing knowledge or skills in the physical, psychological, emotional, social, and behavioral spheres (Wilson, 2017). This means that neuropsychological rehabilitation/habilitation promotes cognitive, behavioral, and emotional changes through a set of practices, techniques, and strategies to minimize the impact of these conditions on the performance of individuals in work, academic, and daily life activities so that the person achieves autonomy and participation in society (Frison et al., 2017; Wilson, 2017).

Therefore, neuropsychological intervention programs should encompass behavior, cognition, and emotion as intrinsic factors (Ben-Yishay, 1996). Neuropsychological interventions focused on the use of strategies that improve cognitive, social, and personality aspects have gained prominence since World War I, through the works of Kurt Goldstein (1942), a German neurologist and psychiatrist, who found these aspects to be fundamental for the patient to return to their daily activities.

Prigatano (2005) even emphasizes that addressing emotional issues in neuropsychological intervention appears as a strong component of success throughout treatment. The patient greatly benefits when they learn to develop coping strategies, when they deal better with their cognitive difficulties and begin to develop feelings of self-compassion, as they become more resilient and experience fewer symptoms of anxiety and depression (Cicerone et al. 2011; Joormann, 2018; Prigatano, 2005). Such aspects are equally relevant in working with children and adolescents.

For this reason, the therapist should consider emotional and psychosocial aspects since cognitive impairment affects the child's quality of life and interferes with their daily routine (Carvalho et al., 2017). Joormann (2018) highlights that cognition plays an important role in the production of emotions and that the way of thinking is capable of modulating emotion. Therefore, if the patient perceives their difficulties and believes they cannot perform certain school activities or their daily tasks, they may involuntarily develop negative self-deprecating thoughts and pessimistic ideas.

Therefore, considering the process of neuropsychological rehabilitation/habilitation, it is important to emphasize that thoughts, emotions, cognitive, behavioral, and social skills are also targets of intervention to fulfill the purpose of promoting active changes in the person who has become incapable or who has started to present difficulties in any of the aforementioned aspects (Wilson, 2017). Therefore, the therapist needs to be attentive in identifying which thoughts are dysfunctional and what their consequences are in the person's life so that it is possible to choose the techniques and strategies to minimize the impact of these conditions on the performance of individuals in work, academic, and daily life activities so that the person achieves autonomy and participation in society (Frison et al., 2017; Wilson, 2017).

Neuropsychological Intervention of Cognitive and Emotional Skills

The patient's complaints and/or those of their relatives, combined with a neuropsychological evaluation, are taken as the starting point for stimulation and/or rehabilitation (Rodrigues et al., 2017). The neuropsychological evaluation is a procedure that provides information about the ability and/or difficulty of concentration, inhibition, cognitive flexibility, perception, reasoning, language, learning skills, memory performance, and behavioral and emotional aspects through neuropsychological tests and techniques. In addition, the evaluation allows an investigation of family and environmental aspects to better understand the child's characteristics (Antunes et al., 2018).

The neuropsychological evaluation should be comprehensive enough to satisfy the objectives of the investigation and also report on the abilities and limitations of each patient. Therefore, the neuropsychologist must be technical, flexible, curious, creative, and empathetic so that, at the end of the evaluation, they can describe accurate information about the cognitive and emotional functioning of the patient and clarify how this impacts their experiences and behaviors (Lezak et al., 2012). For this, the neuropsychologist needs to have a high level of knowledge about behavior, neuroscience, cognitive functions, different clinical conditions, and the instruments and forms of assessment (Miller, 2018). Although experience with clinical practice is very important in developing a professional's clinical skills, it is essential that these skills are also built from the knowledge of evidence-based practices available in scientific publications. This type of knowledge allows for shaping the professional's clinical reasoning and consequently guiding their conduct (Bowden, 2017). In this way, it will be possible to define each patient's problem, outline more appropriate interventions and establish goals and strategies to promote the necessary changes in the person's life (Gorske & Smith, 2009). More about neuropsychological assessment and its role in outlining intervention in childhood can be found in Chap. 1 of this work.

Several professionals often carry out cognitive stimulation. For this reason, the actions chosen by the professional must be explicit due to the transparency in communication between other professionals who may be treating the same patient. In addition, during the entire intervention process, the implemented strategies are evaluated to check which ones worked and which ones need to be changed. This practice also helps family members and caregivers who live with the child, as they can more easily identify the most effective actions. Moreover, this type of conduct helps to clearly report which results are being achieved and indicates which objectives need to be reformulated or maintained (Gindri et al., 2012; Heugten, 2017).

As we can see, the practice of neuropsychological intervention is a great challenge in terms of promoting neuroplasticity. At all times the professional must keep in mind which experiences to provide to the patient in the intervention environment, thinking about each goal established in the intervention proposal (Evansand & Krasny-Pacini, 2017). This includes the involvement of the child's family or parents, caregivers or people involved in the treatment who need to learn the strategies or ways to deal with the affected person to maximize their performance or improvement process (Hart, 2017). In severe neurological cases such as traumatic brain injury, it is essential for the family to partner and engage in the child's rehabilitation and often parents do not adhere to the treatment, which ends up making it difficult to achieve more promising results. However, it is important to align the expectations of both the child and the family in relation to the possible results to be achieved, as often the improvements achieved are subtle but no less important (Evansand & Krasny-Pacini, 2017). Another great challenge for the clinician is to have flexibility and creativity both in planning and in implementing the chosen strategies, as they do not always work as expected, and there are not enough publications with studies pointing to evidence-based strategies, which serve as a guide for clinical practice (Hart, 2017).

Therefore, from the results of the neuropsychological assessment, the therapist should plan the stimulation of skills starting by establishing meaningful goals for the child in various contexts in which they live, such as school, family, leisure and social relations, with the aim that they feel confident, capable and autonomous

(Rodrigues et al., 2017). The process of planning the session, that is, the establishment of goals, is paramount, as it is the moment when the therapist will negotiate with the patient and their family the goals to be achieved throughout the intervention and, subsequently, define the strategies to be used for the implementation of the objectives (Prescott et al., 2015).

A good way to establish goals and select strategies is to think about what end is expected with the process of neuropsychological intervention, that is, what and how the generalization of learned skills and behaviors to the real world can be achieved. Specifying what changes are desired leads to well-founded choices of strategies that will make such changes happen (Hart & Ehde, 2015). This is why it is indicated to professionals to use evidence-based strategies (Cicerone et al., 2011; Snyder et al., 2015).

The selection of a specific and measurable goal can be directed towards any aspect of the intervention, that is, not only for changes in the patient's cognitive functioning, but it can also be directed towards the parents, teachers, or caregivers of the child. After this goal selection, one must choose the strategies by which the changes will be achieved (Krasny-Pacini et al., 2017).

Although there are several reasons for referring to child intervention, in general, these interventions are most often requested in cases of traumatic brain injury, learning disorders, or Attention Deficit Hyperactivity Disorder (ADHD), usually with a focus on improving executive functions, motor skills, and behavioral management. Different strategies can be used, such as metacognitive approaches, cognitive training, computerized training, psychoeducation, and behavior maintenance (Evans et al., 2014; Ratanen et al., 2018).

Metacognitive approaches aim to promote declarative knowledge about the learning strategies that the individual uses to solve problems. That is, they stimulate skills related to self-regulation, increasing the child's awareness of their own cognitive functioning (Fernandez-Duque et al., 2000). In addition, metacognition is related to academic skills in reading, writing, and math and consequently supports academic performance (Maras et al., 2017).

Another method that can be used in the neuropsychological intervention process, but should not be used alone, is training-specific processes. This intervention modality has shown good results. However, these are limited only to the specific function or skill trained, be it reading, writing, math, or memory and attention functions. That is, it hardly allows generalization to other skills, both academic and behavioral and cognitive (Cicerone et al., 2011). Despite these issues, specific cognitive training in attention, memory, executive functions, and language plays an important role in remedying deficits in these areas. It has positive effects on the use of compensatory strategies (Barbosa, 2015).

There are evidence-based training programs to stimulate specific skills, among them:

- *Pay Attention!*, which aims to remedy difficulties in sustained, selective, alternating, and divided attention skills, both auditory and visual (Barbosa et al., 2018; Sohlberg, & Mateer, 2001).

- *Cogmed*, a computerized program specifically used for working memory training (Klingberg et al., 2005).
- *Promote-Children*, which aims at training social skills (Falcão & Bolsoni-Silva, 2016).

Also, some programs integrate psychoeducation, training in specific functions, and metacognition for use in educational contexts. Some of these programs can also be adaptable for the clinical context. The reader can refer to Chap. 9 of this book for a little more about this type of program and even to learn about Brazilian products and productions in the area, which deserve international visibility.

Ferrari et al. (2012) suggest that the therapist can also use games, toys, and other specific resources thinking about their goals to stimulate attention skills, visual processing, processing speed, executive functions, praxis skills, and so on. After all, playing contributes to child development, especially in motor, emotional, and social aspects. Therefore, the market offers several options, such as UNO, Face to Face, Lynx, Pictureka, Connect 4, Detective, as well as songs with specific commands, storytelling, and so on. However, it is important to emphasize the therapist's need to not lose focus of the purpose and function of using strategies like these, as the process of skill stimulation should be structured in a way that these tools are used to achieve the objectives established in the planning carried out at the beginning of the process (Hart & Edhe, 2015). To the interested reader, Chap. 12 of Volume 2 of *Neuropsychological Interventions for Children* will address the use of games and play as strategies in the intervention process.

Given the variety of methods that can be used in neuropsychological intervention, the holistic approach to neuropsychological rehabilitation has been widely adopted, as it has shown promising results due to being more comprehensive and allowing greater generalization to everyday life. Holistic neuropsychological rehabilitation programs include a varied combination of cognitive rehabilitation, psychoeducation, and psychosocial support, and, therefore, advocate that the developmental needs of the child and the family should be met taking into account the cognitive, emotional, social, and functional aspects of the child's development (Ratanen et al., 2018).

Beyond specific strategies, within the process of neuropsychological intervention, the use of techniques from psychotherapeutic approaches is appropriate, such as those derived from cognitive-behavioral therapy and behavior analysis. Usually, these techniques are used to promote in the child favorable attitudes, assertive communication, behavioral management in the face of frustrations, modification of cognitions and dysfunctional behaviors (Joorman, 2018; Petersen & Wainer, 2011).

Ways to Track the Results Achieved

Tracking the results achieved is essential both during the intervention and at the end of it. In addition to assisting the therapist in adjusting goals and strategies used, it communicates the child's progress to the child themselves and their family and other professionals who are also monitoring them (Heugten, 2017). One way to track the patient's progress throughout the intervention is to use tasks or neuropsychological assessment instruments punctually, according to what is being worked on with the child during the sessions. Instruments or tasks that assess specific functions, such as attention, memory, academic skills, language, executive functions (Fonseca et al., 2016; Seabra & Dias, 2012a, b; Seabra et al., 2013), behavioral scales (Thorell & Nyberg, 2008; Trevisan & Seabra, 2018), or even clinical observation can be used to verify whether the established goal was achieved or not (Gindri et al., 2012).

Reviewing the Route—General Tips for Therapists

- **Child rehabilitation** is a type of intervention that promotes cognitive, behavioral, and emotional changes through a set of practices, techniques, and strategies to minimize the impact of these conditions on the performance of individuals in work, academic, and daily life activities so that the person achieves autonomy and participation in society.
- **Neuropsychological assessment** allows for defining each patient's cognitive and behavioral profile, outlining more appropriate interventions, and establishing goals and strategies for promoting the necessary changes in a person's life.
- The **strategies** are better selected when there is clarity about which changes are intended to be achieved (goal setting). Use evidence-based strategies as much as possible.
- **Evaluate** constantly whether the established goals were achieved and if the strategies are promoting tangible results.

Final Considerations

This chapter aimed to point out some challenges and important characteristics that therapists working with child rehabilitation need to have and also guide therapists regarding planning, goal selection and strategies, and monitoring in neuropsychological intervention. Thus, it is possible to see how much the therapist plays a fundamental role in neuropsychological intervention and how complex this is. Therefore, each intervention plan should be carried out individually, according to the complaints and demands of each child, as well as being based on the results found in the neuropsychological evaluation. In addition, the importance of parent and caregiver involvement is highlighted at this stage and throughout the intervention process.

There are several techniques and stimulation strategies that can be used in combination, but the effectiveness of the intervention also will depend on the engagement of the child and involved family members, frequency and duration of sessions, and environmental adjustments. It is up to the therapist to have skill in choosing evidence-based strategies and using other complementary ones in a way that understands what works with their patient, monitoring whether the initially established goals are being achieved or not.

References

Abrisqueta-Gomez, J. (2012a). Reabilitação cognitiva baseada em evidências científicas: recomendações para a prática clínica. In J. Abrisqueta-Gomez (Ed.), *Reabilitação Neuropsicológica: abordagem interdisciplinar e modelos conceituais na prática clínica* (pp. 137–153). Artmed.

Abrisqueta-Gomez, J. (2012b). Reabilitação Neuropsicológica interdisciplinar: reflexões sobre a relevância da abordagem holística. In J. Abrisqueta-Gomez (Ed.), *Reabilitação Neuropsicológica: abordagem interdisciplinar e modelos conceituais na prática clínica* (pp. 19–34). Artmed.

Antunes, A. M., Júlio-Costa, A., & Malloy-Diniz, L. F. (2018). Como explorar a queixa clínica na avaliação neuropsicológica de pré-escolares? In N. M. Dias & A. G. Seabra (Eds.), *Neuropsicologia com pré-escolares: avaliação e intervenção* (pp. 61–80). Pearson.

Barbosa, D. L. F., Miranda, M. C., & Bueno, O. F. A. (2018). *Pay Attention! Programa do treinamento dos processos atencionais para crianças*. Hogrefe.

Barbosa, D. L. F. (2015). Transtorno do Déficit de Atenção e Hiperatividade/Intervenções Cognitivas e Comportamentais. In E. C. Miotto (Ed.), *Reabilitação Neuropsicológica e Intervenções Comportamentais* (pp. 61–80). Roca.

Ben-Yishay, Y. (1996). Reflections on the evolution of the therapeutic milieu concept. *Neuropsychological Rehabilitation, 6*(4), 327–343. https://doi.org/10.1080/713755514

Bowden, S. C. (2017). Why do we need evidence-based neuropsychological practice? In S. C. Bowden (Ed.), *Neuropsychological assessment in the age of evidence-based practice* (pp. 1–14). Oxford University Press.

Cardoso, C. O., Dias, N. M., Seabra, A. G., & Fonseca, R. P. (2017). Program of neuropsychological stimulation of cognition in students: Emphasis on executive functions—Development and evidence of content validity. *Dementia e Neuropsychologia, 11*(1), 88–99. https://doi.org/10.1590/1980-57642016dn11-010013

Carvalho, J. C. N., Mônego, N., Guimarães, E. R., Bertagnolli, A. C., & Kristensen, C. H. (2017). Reabilitação Neuropsicológica e técnicas em psicoterapia cognitivo-comportamental. In D. R. Fontoura, L. Tisser, O. Bueno, S. Bolognani, & T. Frison (Eds.), *Teoria e Prática na Reabilitação Neuropsicológica* (pp. 109–128). Vetor Editora.

Cicerone, K. D., Langenbahn, D. M., Braden, C., Malec, J. F., Kalmar, K., Fraas, M., Felicetti, T., Laatsch, L., Harley, J. P., Bergquist, T., Azulay, J., Cantor, J., & Ashman, T. (2011). Evidence-based cognitive rehabilitation: Updated review of literature from 2003 through 2008. *Archives of Physical Medicine Rehabilitation, 92*, 519–530. https://doi.org/10.1016/j.apmr.2010.11.015

Diamond, A. (2015). Research that helps move us closer to a world where each child thrives. *Research in Human Development, 12*(3–4), 288–294. https://doi.org/10.1080/15427609.2015.1068034

Evans, S. W., Owens, J. S., & Bunford, N. (2014). Evidence-based psychosocial treatments for children and adolescents with attention-deficit/hyperactivity disorder. *Journal of Clinical Child & Adolescent Psychology, 43*(4), 527–551. https://doi.org/10.1080/15374416.2017.1390757

Evansand, J. J., & Krasny-Pacini, A. (2017). Goal setting in rehabilitation. In B. Wilson, J. Winegardner, C. M. van Heugten, & T. Ownsworth (Eds.), *Neuropsychological rehabilitation: The international handbook* (pp. 49–58). Routledge.

Falcão, A. P., & Bosloni-Silva, A. T. (2016). *Promove-Crianças: treinamento de habilidades sociais: promovendo melhores interações sociais e prevenindo problemas de comportamento.* Hogrefe.

Fernandez-Duque, D., Baird, J., & Posner, M. (2000). Awareness and metacognition. *Consciousness and Cognition, 9*, 324–326. https://doi.org/10.1006/ccog.2000.0449

Ferrari, R., Alencar, G. B., & Viana, D. V. (2012). Análise das produções literárias sobre o uso do brinquedo terapêutico nos procedimentos clínicos infantis. *Revista Eletrônica Gestão & Saúde, 3*(2), 381–394. https://doi.org/10.18673/gs.v3i2.24281

Ferreira, S. B. (2012). Reabilitação neuropsicológica infantil: pressupostos e instrumentos. In L. Caixeta & S. B. Ferreira (Eds.), *Manual de neuropsicologia: dos princípios à reabilitação* (pp. 385–389). Atheneu.

Fonseca, R. P., Prando, M., & Zimmermann, N. (2016). *Tarefas para avaliação neuropsicológica: avaliação de linguagem e funções executivas em crianças.* Memnon.

Frison, T., Tisser, L., Fontura, D. R., Bolognani, S., & Bueno, O. (2017). Reabilitação neuropsicológica: fatos e fantasias. In D. R. Fontura, L. Tisser, O. Bueno, S. Bolognani, & T. Frison (Eds.), *Teoria e prática na reabilitação neuropsicológica* (pp. 11–19). Vetor Editora.

Gindri, G., Frison, T. B., Oliveira, C. R., Zimmermann, N., Netto, T. M., Landeira-Fernandez, J., Parente, M. A. M. P., Ferré, P., Joanette, Y., & Fonseca, R. P. (2012). Métodos em reabilitação neuropsicológica. In J. Landeira-Fernandez & S. S. Fukusima (Eds.), *Métodos em neurociência* (pp. 309–341). Manole.

Goldstein, K. (1942). *After-effects of brain injuries in war: Their evaluation and treatment.* Grune and Stratton.

Gorske, T. T., & Smith, S. R. (2009). Collaborative information gathering. In T. T. Gorske & S. R. Smith (Eds.), *Collaborative therapeutic neuropsychological assessment* (pp. 45–56). Springer.

Hart, T. (2017). Challenges in the evaluation of neuropsychological rehabilitation effects. In B. Wilson, J. Winegardner, C. M. van Heugten, & T. Ownsworth (Eds.), *Neuropsychological rehabilitation: The international handbook* (pp. 559–568). Routledge.

Hart, T., & Ehde, D. M. (2015). Defining the treatment targets and active ingredients of rehabilitation: Implications for rehabilitation psychology. *Rehabilitation Psychology, 60*(2), 126–135. https://doi.org/10.1037/rep0000031

Heugten, C. M. (2017). Outcome measures. In B. Wilson, J. Winegardner, C. M. van Heugten, & T. Ownsworth (Eds.), *Neuropsychological rehabilitation: The international handbook* (pp. 537–546). Routledge.

Joorman, J. (2018). Is the glass half empty or half full and does it even matter? Cognition, emotion, and psychopathology. *Journal Cognition and Emotion*, 1–6. https://doi.org/10.1080/02699931.2018.1502656

Klingberg, T., Fernell, E., Olesen, P., Johnson, M., Gustafsson, P., Dahlstrom, K., Gillberg, C. G., Forssberg, H., & Westerberg, H. (2005). Computerized training of working memory in children with ADHD—A randomized, controlled trial. *Journal of American Academy of Child & Adolescent Psychiatry, 44*(2), 177–186. https://doi.org/10.1097/00004583-200502000-00010

Krasny-Pacini, A., Limond, J., & Chevignard, M. (2017). Rehabilitation in executive function. In B. Wilson, J. Winegardner, C. M. van Heugten, & T. Ownsworth (Eds.), *Neuropsychological rehabilitation: The international handbook* (pp. 6–16). Routledge.

Lezak, M. D., Howieson, D. B., Bigler, E. D., & Tranel, D. (2012). *Neuropsychological assessment* (5th ed.). Oxford University Press.

Maras, K., Gamble, T., & Brosnan, M. (2017). Supporting metacognitive monitoring in mathematics learning for young people with autism spectrum disorder: A classroom-based study. *Autism*, 1–11. https://doi.org/10.1177/1362361317722028

Miller, E. (2018). Some basic principles of neuropsycjological assessment. In J. R. Crawford, D. M. Parker, & W. W. McKinlay (Eds.), *A handbook of neuropsychological assessment* (pp. 7–20). New York.

Petersen, C. S., & Wainer, R. (2011). *Terapias Cognitivo-Comportamentais para crianças e adolescentes: ciência e arte*. Artmed.

Prescott, S., Fleming, J., & Doig, E. (2015). Goal setting approaches and principles used in rehabilitation for people with acquired brain injury: A systematic scoping review. *Brain Injury, 29*(13–14), 1515–1529. https://doi.org/10.3109/02699052.2015.1075152

Prigatano, G. P. (2005). A history of cognitive rehabilitation. In P. W. Halligan & D. T. Wade (Eds.), *Effectiveness of rehabilitation for cognitive deficits* (pp. 3–10). Oxford University Press.

Ratanen, K., Vierikko, E., & Nieminen, P. (2018). Effects of the Exat neuropsychological multilevel intervention on behavior problems in children with executive function déficit. *Cognition and neurosciences, 59*, 483–495. https://doi.org/10.1111/sjop.12468

Rodrigues, J. C., Wagner, G. P., & Holderbaum, C. S. (2017). Contribuições da avaliação neuropsicológica para o planejamento de programas de reabilitação. In D. Fontura, L. Tisser, O. Bueno, S. Bolognani, & T. Frison (Eds.), *Teoria e prática na reabilitação neuropsicológica* (pp. 31–48). Vetor Editora.

Seabra, A. G., & Dias, N. M. (2012a). *Avaliação Neuropsicológica e Cognitiva: atenção e funções executivas*. Memnon.

Seabra, A. G., & Dias, N. M. (2012b). *Avaliação Neuropsicológica e Cognitiva: linguagem oral*. Memnon.

Seabra, A. G., Dias, N. M., & Capovilla, F. C. (2013). *Avaliação Neuropsicológica e Cognitiva: leitura, escrita e aritmética*. Memnon.

Snyder, H. R., Miyake, A., & Hankin, B. L. (2015). Advancing understanding of executive function impairments and psychopathology: Bridging the gap between clinical and cognitive approaches. *Frontiers in Psychology, 6*(328), 1–24. https://doi.org/10.3389/fpsyg.2015.00328

Sohlberg, M. M., & Mateer, C. A. (2001). *Attention process training test*. Lash.

Trevisan, B. T., & Seabra, A. G. (2018). *Inventário de funções executivas e regulação infantil (IFERI) para pais ou responsáveis e professores*.

Thorell, L. B., & Nyberg, L. (2008). The Childhood Executive Functioning Inventory (CHEXI): A new rating instrument for parents and teachers. *Developmental Neuropsychology, 33*, 536–552. https://doi.org/10.1080/87565640802101516

Wilson, B. A. (2017). The development of neuropsychological rehabilitation: An historical examination of theoretical and practical issues. In B. A. Wilson, J. Winegardner, C. M. van Heugten, & T. Ownsworth (Eds.), *Neuropsychological rehabilitation: The international handbook* (pp. 6–16). Routledge.

Chapter 6
Specificities of the Report and Recurring Inquiries Regarding the Feedback of the Results of the Child Neuropsychological Evaluation

Hosana Alves Gonçalves, Bruna Evaristo Scheffer, and Flavia dos Passos Fonseca

Providing feedback on the neuropsychological evaluation is one of the last steps of this investigation process, which involves different methods, as discussed in Chap. 1. In cases of neuropsychological evaluation of children, usually the referral source is the school, the educational psychologist (or other professionals related to learning), the psychologist, the pediatrician, or the neurologist. Thus, in addition to providing feedback on the results to the child's guardians, it is extremely important that the neuropsychologist contacts the referral source in order to collect and provide information about the results obtained and hypotheses raised from the evaluation.

Although neuropsychological evaluation is not a practice restricted to psychologists, they commonly use the written communication standards suggested by the Federal Council of Psychology (CFP) in Brazil. Documents from the CFP provide guidelines that enable a framework for organizing essential information to be included in the report. There are different ways of presenting documentary information that vary according to the purpose of the document. This chapter will address aspects related to the neuropsychological report and oral feedback, both forms of returning the evaluation results extremely important and necessary.

In general, complaints are heard about the technical language of the reports, the difficulty in understanding what the reporter wanted to communicate with certain concepts, and the absence of information about the instruments and techniques used in the evaluation, among other factors. There are situations where the report does not reflect the child's real functioning in everyday life. In these cases, instead of clarifying the cognitive and emotional functioning of the child, the report generates confusion for the family and other involved parties.

H. A. Gonçalves (✉) · B. E. Scheffer · F. P. Fonseca
Conectare NeuroPsi, Porto Alegre, Brazil
e-mail: hosana.goncalves.neuropsi@gmail.com; brunascheffer@hotmail.com; flavia.fonseca@acad.pucrs.br

C. O. Cardoso, N. M. Dias (eds.), *Neuropsychological Interventions for Children - Volume 1*, https://doi.org/10.1007/978-3-031-53586-4_6

The main focus of this chapter will be to provide the professional with resources to clarify to parents, the school, and other referral sources the key points in oral (in-person) and written (report) feedback of the neuropsychological evaluation of children and adolescents. In this sense, the points presented may contribute to neuropsychologists being able to plan a clear and useful feedback process for those interested.

Common Doubts About the Feedback Process

It is common that at the time of referrals for neuropsychological evaluation, those responsible for the child may be curious about how and what content will be addressed at the time of feedback. For this reason, from the first contact, there are already many questions about this.

Similarly, referral sources often request "advancements" in relation to what is being identified during the evaluation process. However, the neuropsychologist will not yet have the means to provide information about the child's performance beyond what can be perceived by clinical observation. In this specific case, when the professional communicates that they do not have enough data to provide partial information on the evaluation results, many parents believe that the professional is just following a protocol provided for cases of neuropsychological examination or respecting ethical guidelines and principles of the profession. However, there are technical explanations for this and the protocol to be followed. This is one of the aspects addressed in this chapter. Various other questions may arise related to the content that will be addressed during feedback. Examples of common doubts and their possible answers will be addressed next.

Why Doesn't the Neuropsychologist Give Partial Feedback (Test Results) During the Evaluation Process?

The neuropsychologist uses various instruments to reach conclusions about the current cognitive and socio-emotional processing of the person being evaluated. After a detailed analysis of scores and sub-scores generated by the tests, the professional seeks to identify performance patterns, associations with situational variables, and relation with characteristics of the child's personality, among various other factors. In addition, the result of a single test does not have the power to illustrate the child's overall functioning.

Another reason why it is not possible to provide partial results is that, in general, the raw points obtained by the child need to be converted into standardized scores for correct interpretation. This requires the professional to consult specific normative tables to convert these scores. In turn, the respective tables and scores are not analyzed during the evaluation session. Thus, it is not possible to determine the child's performance and thus provide preliminary results during the evaluation session.

The quantitative results and their interpretations in the report do not correspond only to the child's raw score. On the contrary, what allows the classification of performance as below average, within the average and above average, for example, is the comparison score of the examinee in relation to the normative standards of what is expected for their age range, their type of school, their school year and/or sex.

Is It Possible to Associate the Deficits Observed in the Evaluation with Brain Lesions?

Children and adults with brain injury usually present deficits in various cognitive domains that are easily identified from neuropsychological evaluation (Anderson et al., 2002; Sekely & Zakzanis, 2018). The results of the neuropsychological evaluation can characterize the deficits resulting from the lesions (Karr et al., 2014), in addition to measuring the severity of the injury considering the levels of cognitive and functional impairments of the child (Treble-Barna et al., 2017). In the case of epilepsies, for example, the evaluation can contribute to identifying the lateralization or the location of epileptic foci or even the nature of the syndrome (Wilson et al., 2015a, b). In summary, the deficits caused by brain lesions proven from neuroimaging exams can be observed from the neuropsychological evaluation.

On the other hand, it is not possible to identify a brain lesion from the neuropsychological evaluation. In other words, deficits and impaired performance in the neuropsychological evaluation do not necessarily indicate brain injury. When the neuropsychologist suspects that the impairments are due to neurological changes, he should refer the individual for neurological evaluation and never suggest possible injuries or damaged brain areas based solely on the results of the neuropsychological evaluation. Neuroimaging tests are required for the evaluator to confirm or refute whether there are brain damages that explain the deficit. If the hypothesis is confirmed, the neuropsychologist can associate cognitive impairments with the affected brain areas.

Several factors are related to cognitive changes beyond brain injuries. Cognitive dysfunctions can occur due to stress (Cowell et al., 2015), poor nutrition (Black et al., 2015; Sudfeld et al., 2015), socio-emotional problems (Haft et al., 2016), sleep disturbances (Vaughn et al., 2015), medication effects (Garcia-Amador et al., 2015), among numerous other causes (Linsell et al., 2015).

In the Feedback of the Results, Will I Know If the Child Has a Diagnosis?

During the feedback of the neuropsychological evaluation results, the neuropsychologist may present and investigate his diagnostic hypotheses with the family members. However, this will not necessarily be the central objective of the evaluation (Pureza et al., 2015). The diagnosis that needs to be presented refers to the cognitive strengths and weaknesses that affect the child's functionality. The neuropsychologist will seek explanations for possible reasons preventing the child from meeting environmental demands, such as understanding school texts. These reasons can be the most varied, for example, failures in working memory, oral language difficulty, and severely impaired intellectual level, among many others. In this case, the difficulties in reading comprehension would not be explained by Dyslexia, for example, so the neuropsychologist may not have one of the diagnoses presented in diagnostic manuals, like the International Classification of Diseases (ICD-11) (World Health Organization, 2018) or the Diagnostic and Statistical Manual of Mental Disorders (DSM-5) (American Psychiatric Association—APA, 2014). However, from the results obtained, the professional can develop clinical, home and/or school intervention strategies that will enhance or compensate for the skills identified as impaired, regardless of a diagnosis.

There may be a demand for an intellectual disability (ID) evaluation, which involves the assessment of the intellectual quotient (IQ) from standardized instruments and analysis of the child's functionality and independence. It is common for professionals to suspect ID and then request neuropsychological evaluation to, in addition to evaluating the possible intellectual deficit, clarify the child's cognitive potential. In this case, if the neuropsychologist identifies intellectual and functional decline, then the ID diagnosis should be clear in the report and explained with clarity during the oral feedback, already providing guidance and tips for clinical, home and school intervention.

The Neuropsychological Report

The neuropsychological report represents the completion of the neuropsychological evaluation process. Although there is no fixed structure for the preparation of the report, some information should be present aiming for clear, objective, and useful writing (for a more in-depth review, it is suggested to read Zimmermann et al., 2016).

In general, drafting a report and formulating clinical reasoning about the cognitive and socio-emotional functioning of the child require the neuropsychologist to have in-depth knowledge about the instruments used. From the knowledge of standardized tests, the professional can perform a detailed analysis of the sub-scores that each generates beyond the total scores and use them as a subsidy for understanding the case. This type of analysis can be done in tasks such as the Hayling Test (Burguess & Shallice, 1997; Fonseca et al., 2010), verbal fluency tasks (Montreal Communication Assessment Battery—MAC Battery) (Fonseca et al., 2008; Jacobsen et al., 2016), the Wechsler Intelligence Scales (Rueda et al., 2013; Trentini et al., 2014) among various other tools useful for neuropsychological reasoning.

In addition, the neuropsychologist needs a theoretical basis to interpret the results obtained with the instruments. The conclusion of a report depends on the writer's ability to make a theoretical-practical relationship with each of the instruments (not only the tests but all the other tools used in the neuropsychological evaluation process) and with the clinical observation of the case. More specifically, knowledge about cognitive processing, based on scientific literature, allows the evaluator to associate the test results with the initial demand and what is observed in daily life. Furthermore, theoretical knowledge allows the neuropsychologist to identify the possible explanatory factors of the patient's current functioning.

Basic Contents of the Neuropsychological Report

Regarding the content of the report, it is essential that the ***identification data*** of the evaluated person are complete. This information will not only be useful for identifying the patient, but also for informing which normative tables were consulted in cases of reassessment or referral to another evaluating professional. The child's data (such as age, education, and sex) can also explain a large part of the evaluation results when associated with the evaluation techniques.

Next, the ***demand*** is described. This is the space where information related to the presented problem, the reasons for the initial referral and the request for the document are communicated. From the analysis of the demand, the adoption of some evaluation procedures in favor of others is justified. It is important that the ***instruments*** selected serve as search tools for answers to the initial demand. They should be briefly described in the document with the reference equivalent to the instrument's version. This information will be extremely useful in the case of reassessment.

The evaluation conditions that can interfere and/or explain part of the results should be explicit (both environmental and in relation to the evaluated person) from the beginning of the report. In this way, the reader will read the document already considering the possible reservations arising from these conditions. For example, it is important to report if the child is using medications such as anticonvulsants, neurostimulants or others that directly influence the central nervous system.

In addition to the ***identification***, the ***description of the demand*** and the ***instruments*** used in the evaluation, it is important that the neuropsychologist specifies ***developmental data*** brought by the informants that may be related to the initial complaint, such as a history of fetal suffering, traumatic brain injury (TBI), psychiatric disorders (such as depression, schizophrenia, among others) and family history of cognitive and/or behavioral changes. Again, the importance of knowledge about neurodevelopmental processes is emphasized. It will allow diagnostic hypotheses to be raised from the first contact of the informants with the neuropsychologist.

On some occasions, it can be quite delicate, although necessary, to disclose information gathered in interviews with informants. In the case of making important data collected in the anamnesis explicit, one must always be attentive to the preservation of the confidentiality of information that may compromise both the patient and third parties involved.

Specifically regarding the presentation of the ***evaluation results***, there may be variations. Generally, they appear structured by groupings of techniques and instruments or by specific domains and/or skills. Lichtenberger et al. (2004) describe the advantages of choosing each report writing model. Writing by domains and/or specific skills such as intelligence, memory, attention, executive functions, visuoconstructive skills, or oral language integrates data from different sources and instruments and is indicated for the context of school or learning difficulties.

It is common to have tables and graphs in a neuropsychological evaluation report since, in general, standardized tests that provide quantitative data are used—these are called aptitude or performance tests (Fonseca et al., 2016; Trentini et al., 2016). The use of tables and graphs in reports can cause strangeness to the reader, and the interpretation of these quantitative data will not always be friendly, so it is important that the report writer writes a clear analysis of these scores. When the report is well written, the explanation of these quantitative scores is clear and easy to understand.

In addition to tables and graphs, other types of graphic indicators can be used such as differentiating the font by format (bold, italic) or by color (different colors to signal impaired or adequate performance). These formats can facilitate understanding, since the various instruments used can have different normative references, cut-off points and ways of interpreting that tend to make the reasoning of laypeople difficult. The qualitative analysis of the results obtained in the psychometric tests and clinical observation should always be described to connect all the results.

Regardless of the report style chosen by the neuropsychologist, the writing should be objective and useful to other professionals, family members, and the patient, allowing a better understanding of the results (Kochhann et al., 2016). More specifically, the language of the report should be technical but, at the same time, accessible. For those strictly technical terms, such as *fluid intelligence*, for example, it is suggested that an explanation with more accessible words be presented in parentheses. In this case, the sentence *fluid intelligence skills are better developed in relation to crystallized intelligence* would become more understandable if it were presented in the following way: *fluid intelligence skills (ability to solve problems even without prior learning, based on reasoning) are better developed in relation to crystallized intelligence (knowledge acquired through experience).*

The report needs to be integrative, and its ***conclusion*** needs to come from the relationship between clinical, developmental, and school history information, the comparison between the scores and sub-scores of the instruments used, and the relationship with the cognitive sub-processes involved (Fonseca et al., 2012). In this way, the neuropsychologist will be able to identify and present performance dissociations, that is, the strengths and weaknesses in the cognitive profile of the person being evaluated (Mansur-Alves & Silva, 2015). The report is a tool for ***referral*** and should be useful for planning interventions (Lichtenberger et al., 2004; Zimmermann et al., 2016). Finally, the report must be signed and dated, as the child's cognitive processing can change over time. For this reason, it is said that the validity of the results presented in the evaluation report may have a limited time (Pellini, 2015).

It is quite common for the neuropsychologist to request a reevaluation within a certain period. This is a common practice, especially when one wants to observe the child's progress after starting or changing some treatment. The report can be shared with the psychotherapist, the speech therapist, the doctor, the occupational therapist, the educational psychologist and all other professionals who work in reversing the child's current condition.

The Oral Feedback

The feedback interview is when the professional verbally communicates the evaluation results to those interested. However, beyond communicating the findings, this conversation should fulfill the important role of answering the questions from the requesters in the initial sessions. That is, this is the moment when the professional explains what the results described in the report mean and how they impact the life of the person being evaluated. In this way, referral options can be made feasible and contribute to the decision-making regarding the actions to be implemented.

The specificity of the content returned to the caregivers and other sources can vary; there are questions whose answers are of interest to one but not necessarily to another (Cunha, 2003). Generally, in all cases, it is the neuropsychologist's responsibility to clarify the role of those involved (ex: role of parents and school) in the current situation that the child is in and suggest specific behaviors for each context to change the situation. Similarly, the results and the report's conclusion should be clearly related to the initial objective of the referring source.

It is advisable to start the feedback interview by revisiting the reason for the search and clearly and succinctly pointing out the procedures used to conduct the evaluation. The caregivers will probably be anxious for the results, so beyond the feedback session, this should be a moment of welcoming and empathetic posture with the emotional state of the family members. In addition, unnecessary descriptions of techniques and instruments that can complicate the conversation and divert the focus from the objective should be avoided. In this sense, the use of terms in technical language should also be moderate. To facilitate understanding, it is suggested that results be associated with everyday examples previously brought by the informants and the observations made by the evaluator throughout the assessment sessions.

The professional can also use other strategies to ensure that both parties are certain that the communication of the results was effective. The neuropsychologist can encourage family members to write in their own words what they understood from the assessment results and use metaphors, drawings, and explanatory videos, among other resources. Upon completion, these records can be analyzed so that the professional can ensure that the caregivers did not distort some information, did not omit important facts and understood the reason for the referrals. Considering that psychoeducation is the first step of a rehabilitation plan, materials such as movies, books, and pamphlets with themes related to the patient's functioning/difficulty can be indicated at the time of feedback.

At school, feedback should focus on aspects of learning and behavior in the school context. In addition to explaining the main results, the neuropsychologist must provide tips on strategies that can be adopted, which will favor the child's academic development, including school adaptation. It is important for the professional to give practical tips and, if possible, written materials with intervention possibilities. The international literature has already clearly addressed the role that school plays in child development in relation to the most diverse spheres (Benzing et al., 2018; Vandenbroucke et al., 2018). However, it is common for teachers and school staff to be unaware of the truth of these effects. Thus, it is up to the neuropsychologist to clarify these processes and how they can be worked on in the academic context.

One piece of information already widely described in the literature and should be reinforced with the school community concerns the positive interactions between the teacher and the student. These positive interactions are related to the development of better skills, such as executive functions. On the other hand, negative interaction can have very harmful effects on the child, as it tends to generate high levels of stress (Berry, 2012; Blair & Raver, 2015). Various strategies have been described as useful and applicable to the school context (Downer et al., 2010). Appropriately using this knowledge, the neuropsychologist can contribute to planning the interventions that the teacher will carry out in the classroom.

Common Questions About the Results of the Assessment

Many children participate for the first time in a process of neuropsychological assessment. Specifically in these cases, although the referral sources and other interested parties (as the caregivers) may be aware of the formal procedures of the assessment (such as the number and duration of the sessions), the structure, style, and content of the feedback remain a mystery. For this reason, it is common for various questions to arise after the feedback interview. We will exemplify some of these questions below.

What to Do from Here?

When the results point to deficits in cognitive functioning, it is important to make the appropriate referrals. Therapeutic indications can be the most diverse depending on the needs and functioning of the child. Some factors can contribute to the absence or little response to interventions, such as the level of severity of neuropsychological deficits, cognitive disorders with organic causes, severe intellectual disability, and lack of motivation (Metin et al., 2016).

In general, when it is necessary to confirm, clarify or refute a clinical diagnosis of any developmental disorder or neurological impairment, in addition to the evaluation of the need for psychopharmacological treatment, it is suggested to refer to a psychiatrist and/or neuropediatrician (Shevell, 2018). A referral is made for speech therapy in disorders affecting oral and written communication (Wilson et al., 2015a, b). These linguistic failures may be related to phonological awareness, lexical access, prosody, and all other oral and written language components. Psychopedagogical follow-up is indicated in cases of learning difficulties or Specific Learning Disorder (Rozek & Martins, 2017).

Identifying cognitive dysfunctions caused by emotional and personality factors is increasingly common. Thus, when signs of anxiety, childhood depression and/or other impairments related to emotional aspects are identified, the referral made is for psychotherapy, especially in the cognitive-behavioral approach. There is growing evidence of the effectiveness of Cognitive Behavioral Therapy (CBT) for pediatric psychiatric conditions characterized by impairments in executive functioning, such as Attention Deficit Hyperactivity Disorder (ADHD) (Montiel et al., 2014). In addition, CBT techniques are commonly used in neuropsychological rehabilitation.

If the Evaluation Result Indicated Various Cognitive Deficits, Does This Mean That the Child Will Be Like This Forever or Is It Possible to Change?

In addition to the possible referrals described above, there are cases where neuropsychological rehabilitation is indicated. Usually, those children with neurological disorders or genetic syndromes that cause cognitive underdevelopment are referred for neuropsychological rehabilitation. The process of neuropsychological rehabilitation is presented in more detail in Chap. 2. Also, there are cases where delays or slowness in processing certain cognitive functions are identified and can benefit from systematized cognitive stimulation. When there is a need for stimulation, the neuropsychologist may suggest that the patient be followed by professionals from specific areas for treatment focusing on cognitive functions. For example, there are cases of children and adolescents with learning difficulties due to executive dysfunction. In this case, the intervention would be psychopedagogical but also focusing on the enhancement of executive processes. Changes in the teaching practices of teachers, prioritizing the stimulation of different cognitive mechanisms from classroom activities, can also be indicated, as well as in the psychotherapeutic process and in the examinee's routine.

Suggestions for Systematized Intervention in School

Various published techniques have proven efficacy for the stimulation and rehabilitation of cognition in various contexts, including in school activities (Cardoso et al., 2016). For example, in Brazil, the Program of Intervention in Self-Regulation and Executive Functions—PIAFEx (Dias & Seabra, 2013) was developed for preschool and first-grade elementary school students. It works on stimulating and promoting the development of executive functions and self-regulation. In turn, the Neuropsychological Stimulation Program of Cognition in Schoolchildren: Emphasis on Executive Functions (PENcE) (Cardoso & Fonseca, 2016) is an early-preventive program for elementary school children. Its objective is to stimulate the development of cognitive and metacognitive strategies in the classroom through playful, cognitive and school activities. Interventions in the school environment with these characteristics tend to be attractive and motivating for children (Cardoso et al., 2016; Klingberg et al., 2005).

In addition to these two proposals developed for the school context, there are other methods that can be used both in school and in the clinical context. This is the case with Cogmed (https://www.cogmed.com/), which is composed of three distinct online software programs (according to age range) aimed at increasing working memory capacity. Another possibility is to Pay Attention! It was developed to train the attention of children aged 4–10 years and is part of the rehabilitation program *Attention Process Training* (APT) (Barbosa et al., 2014; Sohlberg, & Mateer, 2001).

Suggestions for Systematic Home Intervention

Some strategies that assist and facilitate the daily life and the psychosocial functioning of the patient and the family are cognitive adaptation and compensatory strategies, which can be recommended along with educational, vocational or community supports (Thorbecke et al., 2014). Regarding systematic cognitive training for stimulation or neuropsychological rehabilitation, there are several programs and websites that provide computerized and/or *online* stimulation activities (Cardoso & Fonseca, 2016). These applications aim to stimulate the most diverse cognitive components through playful strategies and interactive environments (Tourinho et al., 2016). Cards with representative figures, auditory-verbal tasks (Sohlberg, & Mateer, 2001), active games that require body movements, dance and balance, letters, numbers and colors are examples of stimuli used in computerized games (Mossmann et al., 2016).

Final Considerations

The feedback on the results of the neuropsychological evaluation of children is the last stage of this process and ideally should generate a report with information that clarifies the neuropsychological profile and the interference of environmental, neurodevelopmental, and emotional variables in the cognitive processing of the infant. In addition to the written document, it is extremely relevant that the neuropsychologist informs the results of the evaluation in person and orally. In this way, both the caregivers (or referral sources) and the evaluating professional will be more convinced that the results were communicated effectively.

The session of feedback on the evaluation results aims to clarify the current limitations and potentialities of the child, as well as the possible prognosis. On this same occasion, the neuropsychologist will psychoeducate the family and other interested parties regarding the indicated clinical management for the case based on the results. The indications can range from home and school adaptations to neuropsychological rehabilitation/habilitation.

The main aspect to be considered is that the oral and written feedback needs to provide useful information for planning appropriate interventions for that child. This involves knowledge of the neuropsychologist regarding neurodevelopment to integrate data from different sources of information about the cognitive and socioemotional processing of the child (beyond knowledge on standardized tests) and clarity in presenting the results.

References

American Psychiatric Association. (2014). *DSM-5: Manual diagnóstico e estatístico de transtornos mentais* (5a Ed., Nascimento, M.I, trad.). Artmed.

Anderson, V. A., Anderson, P., Northam, E., Jacobs, R., & Mikiewicz, O. (2002). Relationships between cognitive and behavioral measures of executive function in children with brain disease. *Child Neuropsychology, 8*(4), 231–240.

Barbosa, D. L. F., Miranda, M. C., & Bueno, O. F. A. B. (2014). Tradução e adaptação do Pay Attention—um programa de treinamento dos processos da atenção para crianças. *Psicologia: Reflexão e Crítica, 27*(4), 775–738. https://doi.org/10.1590/1678-7153.201427418

Benzing, V., Schmidt, M., Jäger, K., Egger, F., Conzelmann, A., & Roebers, C. M. (2018). A classroom intervention to improve executive functions in late primary school children: Too 'old' for improvements? *British Journal of Educational Psychology*. https://doi.org/10.1111/bjep.12232

Berry, D. (2012). Inhibitory control and teacher–child conflict: Reciprocal associations across the elementary-school years. *Journal of Applied Developmental Psychology, 33*, 66–76. https://doi.org/10.1016/j.appdev.2011.10.002

Black, M. M., Pérez-Escamilla, R., & Fernandez Rao, S. (2015). Integrating nutrition and child development interventions: Scientific basis, evidence of impact, and implementation considerations. *Advances in Nutrition, 6*(6), 852–859. https://doi.org/10.3945/an.115.010348

Blair, C., & Raver, C. C. (2015). School readiness and self-regulation: A developmental psychobiological approach. *Annual Review of Psychology, 66*, 711–731. https://doi.org/10.1146/annurev-psych-010814-015221

Burgess, P. W., & Shalice, T. (1997). *The Hayling and Brixton tests*. Thames Valley Test.

Cardoso, C. O., & Fonseca, R. P. (2016). *Programa de Estimulação Neuropsicológica da Cognição em Escolares: ênfase nas Funções Executivas*. BookToy.

Cardoso, C. O., Dias, N. M., Senger, J., Colling, A. P. C., Seabra, A. G., & Fonseca, R. P. (2016). Neuropsychological stimulation of executive functions in children with typical development: A systematic review. *Applied Neuropsychology Child, 7*(1), 61–81. https://doi.org/10.1080/21622965.2016.1241950

Cowell, R. A., Cicchetti, D., Rogosch, F. A., & Toth, S. L. (2015). Childhood maltreatment and its effect on neurocognitive functioning: Timing and chronicity matter. *Development and Psychopathology, 27*(2), 521–533. https://doi.org/10.1017/S0954579415000139

Cunha J. A., (2003) Passos do processo psicodiagnóstico. In J. A. Cunha e colaboradores (Eds.), *Psicodiagnóstico-V* (5th Ed., pp. 105–140). Artmed.

Dias, N. M., & Seabra, A. G. (2013). *Programa de Intervenção sobre a Autorregulação e Funções Executivas—PIAFEX*. Memnon.

Downer, J., Sabol, T. J., & Hamre, B. (2010). Teacher–child interactions in the classroom: Toward a theory of within—And cross-domain links to children's developmental outcomes. *Early Education and Development, 21*, 699–723. https://doi.org/10.1080/10409289.2010.497453

Fonseca, R. P., Parente, M. A. M. P., Côté, H., Ska, B., & Joanette, Y. (2008). *Bateria Montreal de Avaliação da Comunicação—Bateria MAC*. Pró-Fono.

Fonseca, R. P., Oliveira, C., Gindri, G., Zimmermann, N., Reppold, C., & Parente, M. A. M. P. (2010). Teste Hayling: um instrumento de avaliação de componentes das funções executivas. In C. Hutz (Ed.), *Avanços em avaliação psicológica e neuropsicológica de crianças e adolescentes* (pp. 337–364). Casa do Psicólogo.

Fonseca, R., Zimmermann, N., Pawlowski, J., Oliveira, C. R., Gindri, G., Scherer, L. C., & Parente, M. A. M. P. (2012). Métodos em avaliação neuropsicológica. In J. Landeira-Fernandez & S. S. Fukusima (Eds.), *Métodos em avaliação neuropsicológica* (pp. 266–296). Manole.

Fonseca, R. P., Jacobsen, G. M., & Pureza, J. R. (2016). O que um bom teste neuropsicológico deve ter? In J. F. de Salles, V. G. Haase, & L. F. Malloy-Diniz (Eds.), *Neuropsicologia do desenvolvimento: infância e adolescência* (pp. 53–62). Artmed.

Garcia-Amador, M., Merchán-Naranjo, J., Tapia, C., Moreno, C., Castro-Fornieles, J., Baeza, I., de la Serna, E., Alda, J. A., Munoz, D., Andrés-Nestare, P., Cantarero, C. M., & Arango, C. (2015). Neurological adverse effects of antipsychotics in children and adolescents. *Journal of Clinical Psychopharmacology, 35*(6), 686–693. https://doi.org/10.1097/JCP.0000000000000419

Haft, S. L., Myers, C. A., & Hoeft, F. (2016). Socio-emotional and cognitive resilience in children with reading disabilities. *Current Opinion in Behavioral Sciences, 10*, 133–141. https://doi.org/10.1016/j.cobeha.2016.06.005

Jacobsen, G., Prando, M. L., Pureza, J., Gonçalves, H. A., Siqueira, L., Moraes, A. L., & Fonseca, R. P. (2016). Tarefas de fluência verbal livre, fonêmica e semântica para crianças. In R. P. Fonseca, M. L. Prando, & N. Zimmermann (Eds.), *Avaliação de linguagem e funções executivas em crianças* (pp. 26–45). Memnon.

Karr, J. E., Areshenkoff, C. N., & Garcia-Barrera, M. A. (2014). The neuropsychological outcomes of concussion: A systematic review of meta-analyses on the cognitive sequelae of mild traumatic brain injury. *Neuropsychology, 28*(3), 321. https://doi.org/10.1037/neu0000037

Klingberg, T., Fernell, E., Olesen, P. J., Johnson, M., Gustafsson, P., Dahlström, K., Gilbellrg, C. G., Forssberg, H., & Westerberg, H. (2005). Computerized training of working memory in children with ADHD-a randomized, controlled trial. *Journal of the American Academy of Child & Adolescent Psychiatry, 44*(2), 177–186.

Kochhann, R., Gonçalves, H. A., Zimmermann, N., & Fonseca, R. P. (2016). Como elaborar um laudo em neuropsicologia. In L. F. Malloy-Diniz, P. Mattos, N. Abreu, & D. Fuentes (Eds.), *Neuropsicologia: aplicações clínicas* (pp. 175–192). Artmed.

Lichtenberger, E. O., Mather, N., Kaufman, N., & Kaufman, A. (2004). *Essentials of assessment report*. Wiley.

Linsell, L., Malouf, R., Morris, J., Kurinczuk, J. J., & Marlow, N. (2015). Prognostic factors for poor cognitive development in children born very preterm or with very low birth weight: A systematic review. *JAMA Pediatrics, 169*(12), 1162–1172. https://doi.org/10.1001/jamapediatrics.2015.2175

Mansur-Alves, M., & Silva, R. S. (2015). Exemplo de documento técnico: avaliação de um caso de suspeita de TDAH, 92-101. In S. M. Barroso, F. Scorsolini-Comin, & E. Nascimento (Eds.), *Avaliação Psicológica: Da teoria às aplicações* (pp. 92–102). Editora Vozes.

Metin, B., Roeyers, H., Wiersema, J. R., van der Meere, J. J., Gasthuys, R., & Sonuga-Barke, E. (2016). Environmental stimulation does not reduce impulsive choice in ADHD: A "pink noise" study. *Journal of Attention Disorders, 20*(1), 63–70. https://doi.org/10.1177/1087054713479667

Montiel, J. M., Bartholomeu, D., Armond, G. D., Jacini, W. F. S., Bueno, C. H., Lima, F. F., & Cecato, J. F. (2014). Associações entre medidas de Funções Executivas e TDAH em crianças em idade escolar. *Neuropsicologia Latinoamericana, 6*(1), 13–21. https://doi.org/10.5579/rnl.2013.0158

Mossmann, J. B., Reategui, E. B., Cardoso, C. O., Fonseca, R. P., Viana, M. F., & Barbosa, D. N. F. (2016). *Um Exergame para Estimulação de Componentes das Funções Executivas em Crianças do Ensino Fundamental I*. Trabalho apresentado no XV Simpósio Brasileiro de Jogos e Entretenimento Digital.

Pellini, M. C. B. M. (2015). Elaboração de documentos escritos com base em avaliação psicológica: cuidados técnicos e éticos. In S. M. Barroso, E. Nascimento, & F. Scorsolini-Comin (Eds.), *Avaliação Psicológica: Da teoria às aplicações* (pp. 44–57). Editora Vozes.

Pureza, J. R., Gonçalves, H. A., Cardoso, C., Zimmermann, N., & Fonseca, R. P. (2015). Avaliação neuropsicológica: Bases teóricas e aplicações. In S. B. Barroso, F. Scorsolini-Comin, & E. Nascimento (Eds.), *Avaliação psicológica: da teoria às aplicações* (pp. 237–270). Vozes.

Rozek, M., & Martins, G. D. F. (2017). Psychopedagogists' conceptions of the learning process and psychopedagogical interventions involving university students with disabilities and/or learning difficulties. *Creative Education, 8*(1), 142–155. https://doi.org/10.4236/ce.2017.81012

Rueda, F. J. M., Noronha, A. P. P., Sisto, F. F., Santos, A. A. A., & Castro, N. R. (2013). *Escala Wechsler de Inteligência para Crianças–4ª Edição (WISC-IV): Manual Técnico*. Casa do Psicólogo.

Sekely, A., & Zakzanis, K. K. (2018). Predictive validity of the neuropsychological assessment battery-screening module for assessing real-world disability in patients with mild traumatic brain injury. *Psychological Injury and Law, 1*(4), 1–11. https://doi.org/10.1007/s12207-018-9329-7

Shevell, M. (2018). The role of the pediatric neurologist in the care of children with neurodevelopmental disabilities. *Pediatric Neurology*. https://doi.org/10.1016/j.pediatrneurol.2018.08.004

Sohlberg, M. M., & Mateer, C. A. (2001). *Attention process training test*. Lash.

Sudfeld, C. R., McCoy, D. C., Fink, G., Muhihi, A., Bellinger, D. C., Masanja, H., Smith, E. R., Danaei, G., Ezzati, M., & Fawzi, W. W. (2015). Malnutrition and its determinants are associated with suboptimal cognitive, communication, and motor development in Tanzanian children–3. *The Journal of Nutrition, 145*(12), 2705–2714. https://doi.org/10.3945/jn.115.215996

Thorbecke, R., May, T. W., Koch-Stoecker, S., Ebner, A., Bien, C. G., & Specht, U. (2014). Effects of an inpatient rehabilitation program after temporal lobe epilepsy surgery and other factors on employment 2 years after epilepsy surgery. *Epilepsia, 55*(5), 725–733. https://doi.org/10.1111/epi.12573

Tourinho, A., Bonfim, C., & Alves, L. (2016). *Games, TDAH e funções executivas: Uma Revisão da Literatura*. Trabalho apresentado no XV Simpósio Brasileiro de Jogos e Entretenimento Digital.

Treble-Barna, A., Zang, H., Zhang, N., Taylor, H. G., Yeates, K. O., & Wade, S. (2017). Long-term neuropsychological profiles and their role as mediators of adaptive functioning after traumatic brain injury in early childhood. *Journal of Neurotrauma, 34*(2), 353–362. https://doi.org/10.1089/neu.2016.4476

Trentini, C. M., Yates, D. B., & Heck, V. S. (2014). *Escala de Inteligência Wechsler Abreviada (WASI): Manual profissional*. Casa do Psicólogo.

Trentini, M. T., Bandeira, D. R., & Krug, J. S. (2016). Escolha dos instrumentos e das técnicas no psicodiagnóstico. In C. S. Hutz, D. R. Bandeira, C. M. Trentini, & J. F. Krug (Eds.), *Psicodiagnóstico* (pp. 68–72). Artmed.

Vandenbroucke, L., Spilt, J., Verschueren, K., Piccinin, C., & Baeyens, D. (2018). The classroom as a developmental context for cognitive development: A meta-analysis on the importance of teacher–student interactions for children's executive functions. *Review of Educational Research, 88*(1), 125–164. https://doi.org/10.3102/0034654317743200

Vaughn, B. E., Elmore-Staton, L., Shin, N., & El-Sheikh, M. (2015). Sleep as a support for social competence, peer relations, and cognitive functioning in preschool children. *Behavioral Sleep Medicine, 13*(2), 92–106. https://doi.org/10.1080/15402002.2013.845778

Wilson, J., Aldersley, A., Dobson, C., Edgar, S., Harding, C., Luckins, J., Wiseman, F., & Pring, T. (2015a). The effectiveness of semantic therapy for the word finding difficulties of children with severe and complex speech, language and communication needs. *Child Language Teaching and Therapy, 31*(1), 7–17. https://doi.org/10.1177/0265659014523299

Wilson, S. J., Baxendale, S., Barr, W., Hamed, S., Langfitt, J., Samson, S., Watanabe, M., Baker, G. A., Helmstaedter, C., Hermann, B. P., & Smith, M.-L. (2015b). Indications and expectations for neuropsychological assessment in routine epilepsy care: Report of the ILAE neuropsychology task force, diagnostic methods commission, 2013–2017. *Epilepsia, 56*, 674–681. https://doi.org/10.1111/epi.12962

World Health Organization. (2018). *International classification of diseases 11th revision (ICD).*

Zimmermann, N., Kochhann, R., Gonçalves, H. A., & Fonseca, R. P. (2016). *Como escrever um laudo neuropsicológico?* Pearson.

Part II
Stimulation and Rehabilitation

Chapter 7
Neuropsychological Interventions for Attention in Children and Adolescents

Nicolle Zimmermann and Narahyana Bom de Araújo

The stimulation and rehabilitation of attentional function always occur in an integrated manner with other practices in clinical or school settings. They are part of a therapeutic plan based on a clinical diagnosis and/or problem situation. Before implementing any plan or strategy, these aspects should be clarified and comorbidities should be considered. Among the comorbidities that can influence the definition of the professional's action plan may be symptoms of hyperactivity, intellectual developmental disorder, amnesia, among others. The problem situation refers to the context or task in which the difficulty is experienced.

Although attention is considered a key function for the operation of others, such as executive and mnemonic, multiple factors, such as psychological (metacognition, emotion, and motivation), physiological (hearing, vision, sleep, quality of breathing and feeding) and environmental (stimuli), influence it. Therefore, despite being a basic function of human cognition, interventions for attention are far from being considered simple precisely because they are dependent on these various factors (Cohen, 2014; Fisher et al., 2014; Mahoney et al., 2005).

For this reason, intervention in attentional function should encompass not only neuropsychological aspects but also psychological, environmental, and physiological aspects through a holistic view of the intervention process. The view that interventions detached from the context bring automatic results to individuals' lives has proven naive over the years of scientific investigation on the subject. Thus, this chapter will present evidence-based interventions that should be applied as part of a larger neuropsychological therapeutic process.

N. Zimmermann (✉)
Private Practice, Rio Grande do Sul, Brazil
e-mail: nicolle.zimmermann@gmail.com

N. B. de Araújo
Policlínica Naval Nossa Senhora da Glória, Rio de Janeiro, Brazil
e-mail: narahyana@hotmail.com

C. O. Cardoso, N. M. Dias (eds.), *Neuropsychological Interventions for Children - Volume 1*, https://doi.org/10.1007/978-3-031-53586-4_7

Evidence-Based Approaches to Attention Stimulation

Psychoeducation and Guidelines

Psychoeducation is an intervention that aims to educate patients, families, and schools about topics related to psychology, whether they are clinical diagnoses or constructs and techniques in psychology. Educating individuals about the types and functions of attention is highly desirable and can significantly contribute to the development of metacognition and self-awareness. This technique is part of neuropsychological stimulation programs, such as the Neuropsychological Stimulation Program of Cognition in Schoolchildren: emphasis on Executive Functions (PENcE) (Cardoso & Fonseca, 2016) and the Training of Educators in Neuropsychology of Learning (CENA) (Pureza & Fonseca, 2016), in which each module is started with a psychoeducation section on the constructs worked. Especially in children diagnosed with Attention Deficit Hyperactivity Disorder (ADHD), a study pointed out that these have similar levels of metacognition about attention but some delay in behaviors related to inattention, such as perception of posture, organization of materials, and greater expression of negative behaviors over time. The authors reinforce the need for structured learning and behavioral interventions (Pezzica et al., 2018).

Regarding attention, it is suggested to teach the concepts of the properties of attention presented in the model of executive functions proposed by Diamond (2013), which involves inhibition of irrelevant internal stimuli (thoughts and emotions), executive attention (selection of attention and inhibition of irrelevant stimuli) and inhibition of behavior, as well as effort control (also called controlled attentional processes) and self-regulation (which involves emotion, motivation, and cognition). In addition, it is relevant to illustrate the differences between types of selective, sustained, divided, and alternating attention.

We can understand selective attention as the individual's ability to direct attention to a certain part of the environment while other stimuli around them are ignored. Sustained attention is understood as the ability to maintain the focus of attention on a certain stimulus for a period of time to perform a certain activity. Divided attention is described as the individual's ability to perform more than one task simultaneously, involving more automatic processes (routine tasks) and others more controlled (non-routine tasks). Finally, alternating attention involves the ability to effectively alternate the focus between one stimulus and another (Lima, 2005).

Other assumptions that can be contemplated in psychoeducation for children about attention are:

1. Attention is fundamental for memorization and learning, as it is highly necessary for encoding, the first stage of learning.
2. Anticipation and preparation are important for sensitization and activation of attention.

3. The non-immediate, later response is determinant for the good selection of the attentional response, that is, the impulsive response that does not consider the analysis can be detrimental to attentional performance.
4. Some stimuli attract more attention because they have specific characteristics, such as content, color, shape, and size.
5. Attentional capacity highly depends on motivation.
6. We have the ability to divide attention; however, this capacity is limited.
7. Automatic attention is less demanding of effort when compared to controlled attention (which requires more conscious and intentional attentional effort); controlled attention is more likely to cause fatigue.
8. The existence of preceding, prior memory about stimuli influences the attentional capacity related to them, that is, prior knowledge of the stimulus or content can improve the identification of errors and failures during attentional analysis.
9. Attention is distributed in the given space; therefore, spatial orientation is influenced by attentional aspects.
10. There is attention directed by *bottom-up* processes, which refer to attention conditioned by stimuli throughout human evolution; there is also attention directed by *top-down* processes, which predicts attention that selects stimuli independently and is directed, considered a higher-order cognitive function (Cohen, 2014).

This concept can be presented playfully through games, books, and drawings. An example of this is the psychoeducation book for children about attention difficulties and ADHD by Tisser (2018). In this children's book, two characters (Mr. "Attentional Focus" and Mrs. "Inhibition of Interference") are presented as the key to "taming" ADHD. Beyond this, psychoeducation can also be done with parents and teachers on the subject. In this area, studies on psychoeducation for parents about ADHD predominate, which involves information about the nature and course of ADHD and its main challenges, treatment options, point systems, monitoring of the school day's progress, and anticipation of rules for violation of agreements (Pliszka & AACAP Work Group on Quality Issues, 2007; Barkley et al., 2000). More about specific interventions in ADHD can be found in Chap. 2 of Volume 2 on Neuropsychological Interventions for Children.

Another important intervention for families of individuals with deficits Attentional is cognitive restructuring for parents, which involves working with common parental cognitive distortions regarding the functioning of children in the context of their school performance, non-collaborative behaviors, and demotivation. Psychoeducation is not indicated for reducing symptoms of inattention per se. Still, it significantly aids in reducing behavioral problems and internalizing symptoms, which are important for responding to other interventions (van den Hoofdakker & van der Veen-mulders, 2007).

Self-monitoring of Attention and Performance

Self-regulation strategies can be implemented through self-monitoring of attentional performance using electronic devices or printed forms that monitor the child or adolescent's performance, filled out by them and the school. For example, for self-monitoring of attention itself, the child can record on a form whether they were paying attention each time a sound signal plays on the cell phone or electronic device. For self-monitoring of productivity, the child can record on a form how many exercises they managed to do, how many pages they managed to read, or how many correct answers they achieved at each pre-determined time interval. The effectiveness of performance self-monitoring is still controversial in the literature, as there are results that point in opposite directions with clinical samples with ADHD. Self-monitoring of attentional functioning has better evidence of effectiveness (Guderjahn et al., 2013; Hodgson et al., 2014).

This same strategy can be used by teachers in relation to target behaviors in the classroom. A target behavior record form can be used daily and filled out by the teacher and the student, with a grading of the acquisition level (it can be by grades or by drawn faces that show faces with joy, neutral and sad). These forms can be discussed daily with the child or adolescent. Another proposal along the same lines is for the teacher to adopt continuous monitoring of the child through pre-arranged signals about dysfunctional target behaviors related to inattention, such as not paying attention to explanations or doing another task while they should be doing the class task (for a review, see Eggett, 2013).

Regarding self-monitoring, it is essential to note the role of the family in establishing routines that assist the child or adolescent in attentional functioning. Collaborative work together with the family is crucial for a good outcome. It is common for families to expect the child or adolescent with attentional difficulties to improve their performance alone through their own desire and initiative. Still, in clinical situations such as ADHD, Autism Spectrum Disorder, Specific Learning Disorder, acquired brain injuries or even in child anxiety and depressive disorders, this assumption is a mistake due to the clinical symptomatology presented and the neural bases that characterize each disorder. Patients need support to build the autonomy desired by family members. With the therapist's help, the patient and family build their motivations for the necessary changes, which can be greater support and effort from parents in the right way for the child or adolescent to acquire the desired autonomy (Sibley, 2016).

Behavioral Strategies

Various behavioral strategies have been described as effective for treating attention deficit. Evidence suggests that behavioral interventions are feasible and effective for attention deficit in different contexts, including school and home activities (Fabiano et al., 2009).

The most used interventions from the perspective of cognitive behavioral therapies are problem-solving techniques, reward systems or token systems, and self-instruction training. The problem-solving training aims to develop coping strategies, promotes self-management and self-regulation skills, increases flexibility in choosing alternatives, and reduces trial-and-error responses. One of the most used is the one proposed by Barkley (2002) and includes seven steps: (1) define the problem; (2) identify what the goal is; (3) list the possible alternatives to solve the problem; (4) evaluate from 1 to 10 each alternative, from the most negative to the most positive; (5) select the best alternative and put it into practice, if the chosen alternative does not work, practice the other alternatives until the problem is solved; (6) accept failures and seek other options to solve the problem; and (7) fulfill the plan and evaluate the results. Although these are techniques that encompass executive functions and not exclusively attention, these techniques can play an important role in the regulation of attention and the direction of behavior towards targets and goals.

Another program that includes the problem-solving technique is the Stop and Think Program, proposed by Kendall (1992). This program, in addition to the problem-solving technique, includes self-instruction and social skills training. The child learns four steps to solve the problem at hand. They are: (1) identify what the problem is to be solved; (2) identify the possibilities of solution; (3) choose the most efficient solution to solve the problem; and (4) implement the chosen alternative and evaluate its effectiveness.

Reward systems or token systems aim to reward appropriate behaviors through rewards or reinforcers so that the frequency of the expected behavior increases. This technique initially requires an external stimulus so the child develops intrinsic motivation later. In this system, a list of problems or target behaviors and a list of rewards are developed. As the child emits the desired behavior, they can exchange it for some item from the reward list (Friedberg & McClure, 2004).

Neuropsychological Activities

There are alternatives to pencil and paper neuropsychological activities that can contribute to the stimulation of attention. Neuropsychological activities can be defined as those built based on the theoretical foundations of cognitive neuropsychology and in which the functions stimulated or evaluated are clearly separable. The search for greater purity in terms of theoretical construct is one of the parameters for the differentiation of neuropsychological activities or tasks from other tasks.

The neuropsychological tasks that stimulate attention use paradigms of cancellation of visual stimuli with different levels of complexity of distractors or the number of targets (very similar stimuli among themselves, with a higher level of difficulty; contrasting stimuli among themselves, with a lower level of difficulty). In addition, there is the possibility of inserting, in conjunction with the cancellation tasks, auditory distractors such as noises or sounds. Another type of task used is the recording of viewing or hearing a target stimulus, for example, by pressing a button when the

Target Stimulus: *

-	/	{	*	{	/	?	+
+	}	?	-	/	-	?	/
}	*	-	/	{	*	}	*
/	{	/	+	*	}	-	/
{	-	{	+	-	/	?	-
/	+	*	-	*	}	*	+
+	-	}	*	+	-	/	-

Fig. 7.1 Example of selective attention task

Part A	Part B	Part C
Target Stimulus: €	Target Stimulus: ♦	Target Stimulus: ⌂

ê ∞ ♦ ê € ⌂ € ☼ ♦ ∞ € ∞ ⌂ ê ♦ ⌂ € ⌂ ☼ ê ♦ ☼ € ê

☼ € ☼ € ⌂ ∞ ê € ⌂ ☼ ê ♦ € ∞ ⌂ ê ∞ ☼ ♦ ∞ ⌂ € ∞ ♦

∞ ê ♦ € ê ♦ ⌂ ☼ ê ♦ ∞ € ê ∞ ♦ ⌂ ∞ ê € ⌂ ♦ ☼ ê ∞

Fig. 7.2 Example of an alternating attention task

Target Stimuli: ? +

-	/	{	*	{	/	?	+
+	}	?	-	/	-	?	/
}	*	-	/	{	*	}	*
/	{	/	+	*	}	-	/
{	-	{	+	-	/	?	-
/	+	*	-	*	}	*	+
+	-	}	*	+	-	/	-

Fig. 7.3 Example of a divided attention task

target stimulus is heard or seen by the patient. These paradigms can stimulate selective attention when the target stimulus is only one (Fig. 7.1); alternating attention when the target stimulus is alternated throughout the task at pre-determined time intervals (Fig. 7.2); sustained attention when the activity is prolonged; divided attention when there are two or more concurrent target stimuli (Fig. 7.3).

The Pay Attention! program (Barbosa et al., 2014; Thomson et al., 2018) was designed for children aged 4–10 years, but it is possible that pre-adolescents may benefit depending on the patient's level of functioning. The program has evidence of efficacy in reading for children with dyslexia when attention training was done before reading training. However, there was no transfer to school writing (Chenault et al., 2006). Another study revealed improvements in behavioral and cognitive measures in children diagnosed with ADHD (Tamm et al., 2013). Among the tasks that make up the program are Card Arrangement, House Search, House Search with CD, Arithmetic with CD, and Auditory Tasks. The tasks are performed through auditory stimuli that the patient must listen to and press a button when they identify a target stimulus, cards with drawings of characters that must be categorized according to pre-defined criteria, and three large cards drawn with houses, in which the children must search for objects or cancel items with different criteria established by the manual.

Computerized Training

Computerized training is a process for improving cognitive functioning through practical and intentional instructions. This type of training has the advantage of being an individualized treatment based on the neuropsychological profile of each patient. Computerized trainings have been widely used as interventions for children with attention deficits.

An example developed in a Brazilian context is "Pedro at Camp," developed by Santos et al. (2015). This software aims to stimulate various cognitive functions, including attention (concentrated, selective, divided, and sustained), perception, spatial planning, episodic-semantic viso-verbal memory, working memory, language, and executive functions, in children from the age of five. The software has ten games: reception, accommodation, dining room, river crossing, tree house, forest trail, cave, treasure chest, kingdom of macaws, and tent. Each of these camp locations aims to stimulate different cognitive functions. The tasks present varying levels of complexity; thus, an individualized therapeutic plan can be developed and directed to the needs of each child. The training instruction emphasizes that during the execution of the tasks, it is important for the clinician to make the child stop and think, reflecting on their responses and planning the next action before executing it; therefore, a pause button was implemented in the software. The tasks that most stimulate attention in the software are Dining Room, River Crossing, Kingdom of Macaws, and Treasure Chest. A study used this software in conjunction with other tools to stimulate memory and attention functions in children with typical development and check the effects on phonological and reading skills. The authors found improvement in the performance of the tasks themselves and improvement in other tasks that demand the same construct (attention and memory) but not in phonological and reading skills (Murphy et al., 2015).

Another commercially available software is Cogmed. Cogmed is an online training *course*, which must be performed by a computer connected to the Internet. Although the main goal of this training is to improve working memory, studies indicate that Cogmed stimulates sustained attention and these results can last up to 6 months (Shinaver et al., 2014). The program has three specific software applications by age for preschool children, school-age children, and adults. The training must be supervised by a Cogmed tutor and lasts for 25 sessions with an average of 30–40 minutes. The intensity and level of difficulty of training with Cogmed can be adapted for each user (Chacko et al., 2013).

Metacognition Strategies

Metacognition, including cognitive monitoring or control of cognition, promotes prediction, verification, monitoring, coordination, and control of cognitive operations. Thus, metacognition includes capabilities that allow a person to successfully engage in independent and intentional behavior (Tamm et al., 2014).

In relation to attention, metacognition is described as the knowledge that people have about their attentional abilities (for example: "I can concentrate for almost 10 minutes"), about cognitive strategies (for example: "To concentrate, I have to focus on a certain activity and at the same time ignore other stimuli"), and about tasks (for example: "This task is long, but I can divide it into some parts"). Metacognitive control of attention includes monitoring the direction of behaviors and thoughts and controlling information processing through inhibitory control and resource allocation (Pezzica et al., 2018).

Another strategy is to use "if-then" plans, which specifically state how the individual will achieve a goal. For example: "*If situation X occurs, then I will do Y.*" For this technique, cards containing self-instructions constructed with the therapist or teacher in the clinical or school environment can be used. An example of a self-instruction card that can be constructed with a child who has difficulty staying attentive throughout the class is the following: "If the teacher is giving an explanation in class, then I should strive to pay attention to what she is saying." This strategy has proven more effective than setting goals about attentional functioning (Gawrilow et al., 2011; Guderjahn et al., 2013).

Metacognition has been used as a valuable tool to improve attention in children with ADHD (Alvarado et al., 2011). Studies indicate that self-monitoring procedures are effective strategies for improving academic performance, and students trained to use these strategies to concentrate show greater accuracy in sustained attention performance (Pezzica et al., 2018).

Children with attention difficulties, especially those diagnosed with ADHD, have difficulty internalizing the control of their behaviors from commands. Thus, self-instruction training is an effective technique in children with attention difficulties; as with training, the child learns to direct their thinking to actions, allowing them to remain attentive to their behavior, evaluate and set new goals. Self-instruction training is a guide to external and internal manifest control, as it promotes an inner dialogue that organizes and prepares thoughts and behavior. This technique facilitates the development of appropriate behaviors and the inhibition of inappropriate ones through strategies such as self-control and self-regulation (Ramalho et al., 2011). Initially, the therapist is the model for developing the technique until the patient internalizes the procedure, which promotes the development of the same behavioral control (Lyszkowski & Rohde, 2008).

Final Considerations

The neuropsychological interventions for attention described in this chapter are classic and current approaches that can be used in combination to promote self-awareness (Steward et al., 2017) and attentional performance (Tamm et al., 2013). The use of combined techniques can address a *continuum* of the manifestation of the attentional function in the lives of children and adolescents and give the opportunity to observe the phenomenon of attention difficulties from different perspectives. Such interventions are relevant not only for greater attentional and academic performance, but also for the construction of healthy beliefs about self-efficacy in children and adolescents with persistent attention difficulties.

References

Alvarado, J. M., Puente, A., Jiménez, V., & Arrebillaga, L. (2011). Evaluating reading and meta-cognitive deficits in children and adolescents with attention deficit hyperactivity disorder. *The Spanish Journal of Psychology, 14*, 62–73. https://doi.org/10.5209/rev_SJOP.2011.v14.n1.5

Barbosa, D. L. F., Miranda, M. C., & Bueno, O. F. A. (2014). Tradução e adaptação do Pay Attention – um programa de treinamento dos processos da atenção para crianças. *Psicologia: Reflexão e Crítica, 27*(4), 775–783. https://doi.org/10.1590/1678-7153.201427418

Barkley, R. A. (2002). *Transtorno de déficit de atenção e hiperatividade (TDAH): guia completo e autorizado para pais, professores e profissionais de saúde*. Artmed.

Barkley, R. A., Shelton, T. L., Crosswait, C., Moorehouse, M., Fletcher, K., Barrett, S., Jenkins, L., & Metevia, L. (2000). Multi-method psycho-educational intervention for preschool children with disruptive behavior: Preliminary results at post-treatment. *Journal of Child Psychology and Psychiatry, 41*(3), 319–332.

Cardoso, C. O., & Fonseca, R. P. (2016). *Programa de Estimulação Neuropsicológica da Cognição em Escolares: ênfase nas Funções Executivas*. BookToy.

Chacko, A., Feirsen, N., Bedard, A. C., Marks, D., Uderman, J. Z., & Chimiklis, A. (2013). Cogmed working memory training for youth with ADHD: A closer examination of efficacy utilizing evidence-based criteria. *Journal of Clinical Child & Adolescent Psychology, 42*(6), 769–783. https://doi.org/10.1080/15374416.2013.787622

Chenault, B., Thompson, J., Abbott, R. D., & Berninger, V. W. (2006). Effects of prior attention training on child dyslexic's response to composition instruction. *Developmental Neuropsychology, 29*(1), 243–260.

Cohen, R. A. (2014). *The neuropsychology of attention* (2nd ed.). Springer. https://doi.org/10.1007/978-0-387-72639-7

Diamond, A. (2013). Executive functions. *Annual Review of Psychology, 64*, 135–168. https://doi.org/10.1146/annurev-psych-113011-143750

Eggett, B. (2013). *A review of self management interventions for children with ADHD and implications for education professionals*. Utah State University.

Fisher, A. V., Godwin, K. E., & Seltman, H. (2014). Visual environment, attention allocation, and learning in young children: When too much of a good thing may be bad. *Psychological Science, 25*(7), 1362–1370. https://doi.org/10.1177/0956797614533801

Fabiano, G. A., Pelham, W. E., Jr., Coles, E. K., Gnagy, E. M., Cronis-Tuscano, A., & O'Connor, B. C. (2009). A meta-analysis of behavioral treatments for attention-deficit/hyperactivity disorder. *Clinical Psychology Review, 29*, 129–140. https://doi.org/10.1016/j.cpr.2008.11.001

Friedberg, R., & McClure, J. M. (2004). *A prática clínica de terapia cognitiva com crianças e adolescentes*. Artmed.

Gawrilow, C., Gollwitzer, P. M., & Oettingen, G. (2011). If-then plans benefit executive functions in children with ADHD. *Journal of Social and Clinical Psychology, 30*(6), 616–646. https://doi.org/10.1521/jscp.2011.30.6.616

Guderjahn, L., Gold, A., Stadler, G., & Gawrilow, C. (2013). Self-regulation strategies support children with ADHD to overcome symptom-related behavior in the classroom. *ADHD Attention Deficit and Hyperactivity Disorders, 5*(4), 397–407. https://doi.org/10.1007/s12402-013-0117-7

Hodgson, K., Hutchinson, A. D., & Denson, L. (2014). Nonpharmacological treatments for ADHD: A meta-analytic review. *Journal of Attention Disorders, 18*(4), 275–282. https://doi.org/10.1177/1087054712444732

Kendall, P. C. (1992). *Stop and think workbook.* P.C.

Lima, R. F. (2005). Compreendendo os mecanismos atencionais. *Ciência e Cognição, l6*, 113–122.

Lyszkowski, L. C., & Rohde, L. A. (2008). Terapia cognitivo-comportamental no TDAH. In A. V. Cordioli (Ed.), *Psicoterapias: abordagens atuais* (3rd ed., pp. 716–731). Artmed.

Mahoney, C. R., Taylor, H. A., Kanarek, R. B., & Samuel, P. (2005). Effect of breakfast composition on cognitive processes in elementary school children. *Physiology and Behavior, 85*(5), 635–645. https://doi.org/10.1016/j.physbeh.2005.06.023

Murphy, C. F. B., Moore, D. R., Schochat, E., & Dick, F. (2015). Generalization of auditory sensory and cognitive learning in typically developing children. *PLoS One, 10*(8), 1–17. https://doi.org/10.1371/journal.pone.0135422

Pezzica, S., Vezzani, C., & Pinto, G. (2018). Metacognitive knowledge of attention in children with and without ADHD symptoms. *Research in Developmental Disabilities, 83*(August), 142–152. https://doi.org/10.1016/j.ridd.2018.08.005

Pliszka, S., & AACAP Work Group on Quality Issues. (2007). Practice parameter for the assessment and treatment of children and adolescents with attention-deficit/hyperactivity disorder. *Journal of the American Academy of Child & Adolescent Psychiatry, 46*(7), 894–921. https://doi.org/10.1097/chi.0b013e318054e724

Pureza, J. R., & Fonseca, R. P. (2016). *Programa de Capacitação de Educadores em Neuropsicologia da Aprendizagem* (1st ed.). BookToy.

Ramalho, J., García-Señorán, M. M., & González, S. G. (2011). Auto-instruções: estratégia de regulação atencional da TDAH. *Psicologia: Reflexão e Crítica, 24*(1), 180–185.

Santos, R. M., Prando, M. L., Frison, T. B., & Casarin, F. S. (2015). Pedro no Acampamento – Habilidades Neurocognitivas. CTS Informática.

Sibley, M. H. (2016). *Parent-teen therapy for executive function deficits and ADHD: Building skills and motivation* (1st ed.). The Guilford Press.

Shinaver, C. S., Entwistle, P. C., & Söderqvist, S. (2014). Cogmed WM training: Reviewing the reviews. *Applied Neuropsychology: Child, 3*, 163–172. https://doi.org/10.1080/21622965.2013.875314

Steward, K. A., Tan, A., Delgaty, L., Gonzales, M. M., & Bunner, M. (2017). Self-awareness of executive functioning deficits in adolescents with ADHD. *Journal of Attention Disorders, 21*(4), 316–322. https://doi.org/10.1177/1087054714530782

Tamm, L., Epstein, J. N., Peugh, J. L., Nakonezny, P. A., & Hughes, C. W. (2013). Preliminary data suggesting the efficacy of attention training for school-aged children with ADHD. *Developmental Cognitive Neuroscience, 4*, 16–28. https://doi.org/10.1016/j.dcn.2012.11.004

Tamm, L., Nakonezny, P. A., & Hughes, C. W. (2014). An open trial of a metacognitive executive function training for young children with ADHD. *Journal of Attention Disorders, 18*, 551–559. https://doi.org/10.1177/1087054712445782

Thomson, J., Kerns, K., Seidenstrang, L., Sohlberg, M. M., & Mateer, C. A. (2018). *Pay attention* (1st ed.). Hogrefe.

Tisser, L. (2018). *Por que eu tenho dificuldade de atenção? Crianças entendendo o transtorno de déficit de atenção-hiperatividade* (1st ed.). Sinopsys Editora.

van den Hoofdakker, B. J., & van der Veen-mulders, L. (2007). Effectiveness of behavioral parent training for children with ADHD in routine clinical practice: A randomized controlled study. *Journal of the American Academy of Child & Adolescent Psychiatry, 46*(10), 1263–1271. https://doi.org/10.1097/chi.0b013e3181354bc2

Chapter 8
Stimulation and Neuropsychological Rehabilitation of Memory

Mariana Abuhamad

We have some conceptual problems not so easy to solve when it comes to memory. This is because we have one term but not only one definition. In addition, we have the term "learning" and its similar definitions. Are these really different things or different aspects of the same thing? Cohen (1997, p. 11) describes learning as "the process of acquiring new information" and memory as "the consolidation and retention of the information acquired." It seems that memory and learning are mixed concepts under large-scale analysis, and it is very difficult to put an end to countless definitions, especially because each of these concepts is an arrangement of processes and new concepts.

What is known so far is that there are many ways to define memory and learning and that for the neuropsychology professional it is extremely important to adopt one or more models to define the function, as the constructs (such as their alterations) need to be understood to be rehabilitated. Working with a cognitive process model helps therapists organize neuropsychological rehabilitation activities, evaluation, and treatment practice. For this reason, this chapter aims to discuss some conceptual definitions of memory and learning and present strategies to control memory difficulties that, despite not being specific from interventions with children and adolescents, are of great value and little understood in terms of efficacy up to the present moment. Moreover, it points out activities to stimulate memory for children and adolescents based on the argument that learning difficulties during childhood and adolescence may be associated with various memory problems, which should be the focus of evaluation and intervention. Finally, evidence-based interventions for this population will be presented.

M. Abuhamad (✉)
Cognos, Curitiba, Brazil
e-mail: mariabuhamad@gmail.com

C. O. Cardoso, N. M. Dias (eds.), *Neuropsychological Interventions for Children - Volume 1*, https://doi.org/10.1007/978-3-031-53586-4_8

Theories About Memory and Learning

Memory and learning are similar and can be easily confused. For authors Miller and Blasik (2010), memory is the ability to recall past events and information, while learning is the process of linking memories with new experiences. However, they point out that memory is essential for learning and is dependent on it. In other words, the more information is stored and can be accessed in memory, the easier it is to link the information between memories, thus facilitating learning.

There are three stages of memory and subsequent learning: encoding, storage, and recall. Encoding involves the processing of information that will be stored in memory; it is the initial stage of memory, the level of analysis performed on the material to be remembered, where remembering a verbal material depends on the encoding of phonological features while remembering visual information depends on the encoding of its graphic representations. Storage implies the consolidation of new information with the information already stored previously in memory; that is, it refers to the transfer of transient memory to a form of permanent retention. Storage can be interrupted when there is a *retroactive interference,* which is the interference in learning new information due to the presentation of subsequent learning material, or when there is a *proactive interference*, which is the interruption in memory due to the presentation of learning material prior to memorizing the new stimulus. Finally, recall is the conscious act of accessing memories or automatically executing learned behaviors (Miller, 2007; Miller & Blasik, 2010; Sohlberg & Mateer, 2011).

Various systems and structures in the brain influence different aspects of memory. The hippocampus, the para-hippocampal gyrus, the entorhinal cortices, and deep bilateral structures in the frontal lobes are decisive for learning. The amygdala and the mammillary body are considered crucial for memories with emotional meaning. The frontal lobes have been investigated as having a very important role in the distribution of attention and the organization of memories, both in time labeling and source control. There is still much to be learned about the neurocircuits of memory; however, in general, structures of the bilateral medial temporal lobe, the hippocampus in particular, and the frontal lobes are the structures most widely involved with the processes of storage and retrieval of information (Muller et al., 2018; Smith, 2014; Grady, 1999; Stuss & Benson, 1986).

Overview of Memory Systems

The human memory system can be fractionated into several subsystems based on the temporal nature of the information. In this chapter, the subsystems will be described according to two perspectives: the perspective of cognitive neuroscience and the perspective of school neuropsychology (a specialty of neuropsychology in the United States).

Organization of Memory Subsystems According to Cognitive Neuroscience

Sensory Memory

Sensory memory is associated with perception and is the ability to briefly retain visual, auditory, or tactile perception after the removal of the original stimulus. The sensory impression is ephemeral, lasting less than 2 s. Sensory memory is a basic and important part of memory, but it is not a construct directly measured (Baddeley, 2004).

Short-Term Memory and Working Memory

Short-term memory is historically used to describe all temporary memories that occur subsequent to sensory memory (Atkinson & Shiffrin, 1968). However, the development of more articulated theories about working memory shows that short-term memory is an aspect of the working memory system. The difference is that short-term memory is best used to describe temporary memories that are simply repeated without transformation while working memory actively involves the transformation of this information via the recruitment of additional attentional resources. Short-term memory is a lower-order process of the working memory system underlying the phonological loop and visuospatial sketchpad.

The most frequently cited working memory model is that of Baddeley and Hitch (1974). This model provides an organized structure for evaluation and intervention and was initially composed of three components. Still, an update by Baddeley (2003, 2004) included a fourth component responsible for transferring the information from working to long-term memory. The model's four components are: (a) the central executive, (b) the phonological loop, (c) the visuospatial sketchpad, and (d) the episodic buffer.

The central executive is responsible for controlling attention to the other components of the model. Specifically, Baddeley (2003) argues that the central executive is responsible for focusing, dividing, and switching attentional resources. The phonological loop has limited capacity and is under the control of the central executive as a "slave" system. It actively maintains rules for problem-solving and learning (Engle et al., 1999). The visuospatial sketchpad, also under the control of the central executive, is responsible for visual and spatial information. Both the phonological loop and the visuospatial sketchpad have short-term storage and information retrieval functions. The final component is the episodic buffer, which updates the stock of information stored in long-term memory, allowing new knowledge to be quickly assimilated or accommodated alongside existing information networks.

Long-Term Memory

At the most global level, long-term memory can be fractionated into two types based on the effort required for recall: explicit (declarative—knowing "what") and implicit (non-declarative—knowing "how"). The explicit memory system requires intentionality and conscious effort to activate working memory and the episodic buffer (Postle, 2007). On the other hand, implicit memory is not intentional; it is automatic and does not require effort to be activated.

Explicit memories are derived from experience with the external world and can be semantic, episodic, and lexical. Semantic memory is the collection of all someone's knowledge about facts and objects; it is broad, complex, and structured. The information can be representational and consistent with the outside world and purposeful and symbolic (Tulving & Markowitch, 1998). Episodic memory includes the storage and retrieval of personal events in a temporal context; it is knowing the what, when, and where of events that are retrieved. For Tulving (2002), episodic memory is the memory system that allows us to consciously experience a past event. Episodic memory is the last to develop in children and is the first to be compromised in adults. Finally, lexical memory is specific for decoding spoken and written language (Martin, 2003); its fluent operation allows for auditory comprehension, oral expression, reading, calculation, and writing. Specifically, the phonological lexicon stores known phonemes used in the comprehension and generation of fluent oral language. The orthographic lexicon stores known graphemes used in the decoding and production of written language.

Implicit memory, also known as non-declarative memory, can be considered procedural memory, as it stores automatic schemas that facilitate other cognitive tasks, skills, and behaviors and includes learning a variety of motor tasks. It may also contain perceptual *priming*, a phenomenon by which a stimulus can stimulate an accurate recall without the individual being aware of this stimulus, in addition to simple behaviors learned through conditioning, habituation, or sensitization (Gazzaniga et al., 2006).

Evidence-Based Interventions for the Treatment of Children and Adolescents with Memory and Learning Dysfunction

The extent of the evidence of interventions in memory and learning in children and adolescents depends on the type of deficit in these skills. There is certainly extensive literature on the treatment of children with learning problems. However, despite advances in theories and assessment tools for memory subsystems, in general, the intervention of these processes is not yet well structured. Below, you will find some treatment protocols based on the evidence in the literature, some approaches to control memory deficits, and suggestions for cognitive stimulation resources.

Next, Table 8.1 summarizes the principles of cognitive stimulation that should be respected in planning a stimulation program that seeks to enhance neural plasticity.

Table 8.1 Principles of cognitive stimulation for intervention planning

Principle	Description	Implications
Specificity	The nature of the training dictates the nature of the plasticity.	During the initial training phase, strive to keep stimuli and contexts as close to tasks as possible.
Interference	Plasticity in response to an experience can interfere with the acquisition of other behaviors.	During the initial training phase, ensure that the training does not address multiple targets simultaneously.
Importance matters	The training experience must be sufficiently important to induce plasticity	Tasks and target behaviors should be relevant and significant to the client.
Time matters	Different forms of plasticity occur at different times throughout the training: High frequency of rehabilitation in the acute stage has been associated with significant improvement in the chronic stage.	Do not assume that the significant opportunity for change ends after spontaneous recovery reaches its maximum.
Age matters	The effects of the intervention are different at different ages: Very young brains (−1 year) have plasticity that is not adaptive; brains of older ages (+65 years) are less plastic than those of young people (1–65 years).	Although young brains show optimal ability to replace function, they have few established pathways to support learning new behaviors. All ages can benefit from rehabilitation, but plasticity will operate differently at different ages.
Use it or lose it	Failure to use specific brain functions can lead to the functional decline of these functions.	Gains require maintenance over time. Consider a schedule for maintaining gains.
Use it and improve	Training directed at specific brain functions can lead to an increase in that function.	Focus on specific and functional targets.
Repetition matters	Induction of plasticity requires sufficient repetition.	Provide large amounts of practice.
Intensity matters	Induction of plasticity requires sufficient training intensity.	Provide intensive practice during the initial acquisition of the target.
Transfer	Plasticity in response to training experience can increase the acquisition of similar behaviors.	Actively promote generalization to similar treatment targets.

Source: Sohlberg and Turkstra (2011)

Rourke's Developmental Rehabilitation Model

The treatment of memory and learning problems in cases with other acquired neuropsychological deficits begins with determining the expected degree of recovery from the acquired loss of function. For cases of memory deficits associated with developmental problems, the consideration to be made is about the current levels of functioning and projected improvement (Rourke, 1994).

Rourke's developmental rehabilitation model (Rourke, 1994; Work & Choi, 2005) is exactly that: it considers the problem's presentation, examines the probability of recovery, and outlines a course of treatment involving the child's academic and social contexts. The treatment begins with a biopsychosocial examination of the child's learning problems, these data being derived from a comprehensive assessment that includes observation, interview, neuropsychological assessment, and medical and neurological data. The next step is to discover the demands derived from the immediate context regarding academic and social functioning. Afterward, the projected demands for the beginning of adult life in the domains of work and social interaction of that child and adolescent are examined, since there is a correlation between academic skills and professional success, as well as social functioning in childhood and social interaction skills and leisure activities in adult life. From these projections, a short and long-term intervention plan is established. This plan is adjusted to the resources available by the family, school, and health systems. In most cases, the optimal intervention plan has to be adjusted to a realistic intervention plan.

This model has four bases of treatment approach: improvement, restoration, accommodation, and compensation. The improvement of functioning is based on the evidence that memory can be improved with intervention (Conner et al., 2008; Dehn, 2008). Restoration is related to the loss of memory function or learning after an injury or neurological insult; its goal is to return the individual to their pre-morbid level of functioning. Thus, cognitive rehabilitation, at this first moment, should be offered intensively until the child can reach pre-morbid levels of functioning. Accommodation is related to the organization of the child's environment to maximize their success, which is quite feasible in school environments in association with individualized educational programs. Finally, compensation includes introducing external devices such as notebooks, voice recorders, calendars, smartphones, and others that the individual can use in their context to compensate for their memory difficulties and their ability to learn.

Specific Memory Interventions

The evidence-based interventions suggested by the literature and presented below can be organized as follows: (a) practice and rehearsal, (b) mnemonic strategies, (c) environmental support and external devices, (d) prospective memory training, (e) expanded rehearsal, (f) use of *priming*, and (g) errorless learning.

Practice and Memory Rehearsal Exercises

This intervention is indicated for all levels of memory problems. The approach of distributed practice through repetition is based on the premise that the more memory is practiced, the more likely it will be retained over time. Intervention plans that include practice and rehearsal should organize intervals between learning and rehearsals, reviewing the material to be remembered from time to time.

Repetition means practicing or repeating something until it is memorized. Mechanical repetition is widely used by the general population. However, those with memory difficulties know that this is not a very good strategy (Wilson, 2009). Mechanical repetition has limited value, but there are other methods of repetition that improve recall. The most used repetition strategy in memory rehabilitation is the PQRST method (from the English acronym Preview, Question, Read, Self-recite and Test) (Robison, 1970 cited in Wilson, 2009). The steps are:

- *Preview*: Preview the material to be remembered (have a general idea of the content).
- *Question*: Before reading the material, ask key questions. (What is the main point? In what year did it happen? How many people were involved?)
- *Read*: read the material carefully to answer the questions.
- *Self-recite*: describe the answers and, if necessary, read again until you can answer all the questions.
- *Test*: test from time to time to see if you remember the information.

According to Wilson (2009), this method gives better results because the formulated questions provide the recall cues. In addition, recall is increased when the learning situation is reestablished at the time of recall. Thus, if the test situation is similar to the original learning, more information will be recalled. In the PQRST situation, the questions are part of the original learning situation and part of the test situation. Finally, another justification for this strategy's effectiveness is that information processed at a deeper level is more retained than information processed at a more superficial level. With this, the PQRST method seems to lead to a deeper processing than the practice of repetition because people have to think about the passage and what they are hearing and reading to complete each step (Anderson, 2004; Wilson, 2009).

Within this approach of practice and memory rehearsal, there are also exercises to stimulate this skill by resorting to structured activities and games to stimulate the function through intensive and repeated training. Some suggestions can be found on the following websites:

Cognos Cognitive Stimulation Activities: www.cognos.vc

Some specific games for memory stimulation that cover the age range of 5–16 years will be mentioned below:

- Operating Sequences: In this game the participant is asked to pay attention to a sequence of cards that may initially contain three stimuli (the number of stimuli can be increased or decreased according to the participant's performance), the stimuli can be: animals, numbers, letters or colors. In each round a new stimulus will be added to the previous sequence and the participant should report the last three stimuli only. For example, the sequence of numbers presented is 7–9–2, then the patient repeats: 7–9–2. Then, a new stimulus is added: 7–9–2–4, then the patient will respond only 9–2–4 and so on.

- Gala Dinner: In this game a card of application containing a dinner scene is presented to the participant with the following stimuli to be learned: characters' faces, names of each of them, chair colors, position of each character at the table and menu that may contain starter, main course, dessert and drink of each of the characters. After learning this information, a table and cards containing the learned stimuli and other distractors are given to the participant, and he should reconstruct the scene learned on the application sheet.
- Remembering Positions: A card containing fruits distributed in certain spaces of the application card will be given to the participant. After learning time, a response card is given to the child in which they should fit the correct fruits in their respective spaces, according to the application card.
- Moving Objects: An application card, which reproduces a desk, is given to the child, and then they are asked to carefully visualize the objects that were left on top of the desk. Then, cards with objects and office materials are arranged on the table for the child to point to those they recognize were present on the application card.

Idea: www.ideajogos.com.br
NeuroCognition: www.neurocognição.com.br
Stimuli: www.lojaestimulos.com.br
CogMed: www.cogmcd.com.br

Generally, the main target of cognitive stimulation programs with school-age children and adolescents is working memory, precisely because it is considered critical for learning, development of academic skills, planning and problem-solving, in addition to being recognized as a predictor of the level of achievement in math and reading skills (Johnson et al., 2010; Pascoe et al., 2013; Rode et al., 2014). For more information about strategies for stimulating working memory, the book listed in the references of this chapter is suggested: *Working Memory and Academic Learning: Assessment and Intervention.*

Mnemonic Strategy Training

There are mnemonic strategies that we can learn, and with effort to put them into practice, we can remember things more easily. Mnemonics are systems that allow us to remember things more easily. Generally, it can be defined as consciously learned internal strategies that require effort to put them into practice (Glisky & Glisky, 2002; Miller, 2007; Sohlberg & Mateer, 2011; Wilson, 2009). However, they are indicated for those with less memory impairment, as the technique will require the child to imagine, associate, and review the material to be remembered. Once the child is able to generate a mnemonic strategy, they should intentionally identify opportunities for the use of the strategy (Glisky & Glisky, 2002). An example of an artificial strategy is when we use the "knuckles" of our hand to remember how many days each month has: the months of the "knuckles" have 31 days and the months that fall in the "valleys" have 30 days (except February).

Verbal Mnemonic

Other strategies are using the first letters of words in a sentence to remember information in a specific order.[1] *Example:* The names of the planets in the solar system in order: *My Grandma Has Many Jewels and Only Uses Them On Her Neck*: Mercury, Venus, Earth, Mars, Jupiter, Saturn, Uranus, Neptune, and Pluto (currently understood as a dwarf planet). The linking verbs were remembered through a single word:[2] *S E PA PE FI CO AN*: To be, To stay, To seem, To remain, To become, To continue, and To walk. Or, still, to remember the colors of the rainbow: the *CANDLE WILL Turn* (Red, Orange, Green, Blue, Indigo, Violet).

A variation can be used to remember a list of numbers, like our credit card password. *Example*: we can create a sentence or a word in which each word consists of a number of letters corresponding to the numbers to be remembered: 5764: *Mommy* (5 letters) *courage* (7 letters) *was* (3 letters) *here* (4 letters).

The first letter strategies are only useful when the material is well known but difficult to be evoked in the correct order.

- *Why does the first letter strategy work?*

(a) Because the information is being grouped and grouping facilitates recall.
(b) It reduces the number of possible responses.

Another method to improve recall is the creation of stories. Our semantic memory lives in a world of words. It is activated by associations, similarities, or contrasts. Stories provide a scheme or *script* to link or anchor information in our memory. Also, concrete images engage our emotions and sense of meaning, providing a context and cue for the new information (Wilson, 1987).

Visual Mnemonics

It is the remembrance through figures. These can be mental images or real figures. *Example:* We can transform a name into a visual image and remember the image to remember the name. In the case of the name Daisy, just remember the flower with the same name. Also, it can be done through an image that rhymes with the name *Mariana—banana.* That is, an association is made from the image to the name. Also, we can remember certain words more easily if we associate them with gestures. For example, the word baby can be more easily learned if we associate it with the rocking movement.

[1] Strategy known as Acrostic.

[2] When the letters of the stimuli to be remembered are used to form a single word it is called an Acronym.

Environmental Support and External Device

External devices are seen as methods to compensate for a reduction in memory or organizational skills, which means reducing the load on memory or executive functions to allow the child to organize the task more successfully or minimize the harm of the cognitive disorder. Therefore, implementing an external device involves teaching a series of behaviors instead of retraining a process. The device can be used to complete a specific task or in various contexts. Some information about compensations through the use of an external device:

- Compensations are intentional and goal-oriented.
- Compensations are often pre-existing or "normal" behaviors that are adapted in some way to compensate for a problem.
- Compensatory strategies seem to be employed in flexible patterns to adjust to a context; that is, it is important to understand when and where they will be necessary because we will not always have a device exactly thought out and built for the demand of our patient, for this reason we will need to adjust them to the needs of the child or adolescent.
- Compensations are specific to the participant.
- Many compensatory strategies are spontaneous.

How to Select an External Compensatory Device?

The first step is to identify or develop a system matching the child. For this, it is necessary to conduct an assessment of needs. The second step is to appreciate the available options of external devices.

Assessment of Needs

More than conducting a formal assessment, the therapist can request information from people relevant to the individual's environment. One way to match the system to the individual is to assess organic factors (physical and cognitive functions), personal factors (psychosocial and environmental elements) and situational factors (context of use).

- Organic Factors: it is important to understand the child's strengths and weaknesses and that this impacts the ability to use specific devices. The cognitive/learning profile influences the use of the device. For example, using devices with multiple steps in patients with severe memory deficits may not be possible. Also, disorders of motor skills or sensory functions will limit the device alternatives.
- Personal Factors: it is much more effective to work with existing strategies than to develop and train a new habit, as some patients use spontaneous compensation strategies. However, with children and adolescents we will not always find this scenario. In addition, it is useful to identify the child's inclination for behavior

compensatory. The person's previous experience with compensatory strategies will influence their current behavior. Learning about the patient's personal preferences for the external device will increase motivation and agreement to use a system. It is important to understand the preferences for appearance and model, to include the child in the choice of the device, such as its color, size, etc. The level of support available in the environment will also affect the recommendations for an external device. If a client has support from people who can assist them with training and generalization, a sophisticated system that initially requires external assistance may be reasonable.
- Situational Factors: the therapist needs to understand the context of the cognitive problem. They need to have a clear understanding of the problem or the goal that the external device will address. Another important situational factor is identifying which adaptations and strategies have already been tested.

What Are the Options for External Devices?

- Low-tech resources, such as written agenda systems, which include agendas, notebooks divided into sections, notebooks, and electronic calendar and agenda systems.
- Medium-tech resources: Computerized Systems, such as:
  - NeuroPage: http://www.ozc.nhs.uk/ozc-neuropage.asp
  - Timex Data Link Watch: https://www.youtube.com/watch?v=64EAfXsX828
  - Electronic Agenda.
- High-tech resources: smartphones and apps.
- Auditory or Visual Systems: patients who cannot read or write may benefit from using auditory or visual symbols, such as voice electronic organizers and abbreviated speech recorders. Therapists and family members can use symbols that can be used in agendas or daily calendars.
- Task-specific devices: refrigerator pad, GPS, *post-it*, writing/grammar checkers, calculator, etc.

How to Train the Use of an External Device?

Adopting a new habit takes time: many individuals require repetition and repeated opportunities to implement a strategy before it becomes routine. It is common for some success during the initial period when motivation is increased. Afterward, individuals tend to exhibit highs and lows in implementation. Having realistic expectations can prevent us from prematurely abandoning an external device that may have good potential to be effective if the acquisition period and failures in the use of the strategy are planned.

Patience is needed when partnering with caregivers: training the use of an external device demands the involvement of people who interact with our patients in different environments, which requires us to coordinate our efforts between school, family, and the child. It can be frustrating when a program depends on others who do not agree with the organization of tasks.

Like everyone, clients need reinforcement: learning to use an external device when the client has a cognitive disability is a high ambition and can be a frustrating experience. Despite wanting to learn to compensate for a cognitive deficiency, clients are not always motivated enough. It is common for therapists to offer a lot of verbal instruction in the education of a compensatory strategy and little practice in doing the skill. It is essential to provide clear instructions with ample demonstrations.

Prospective Memory Training

Prospective memory refers to the ability to remember to organize intentions (Wilson, 2009), such as remembering homework or future tests and tasks. In this type of training, repeated prospective memory tasks are administered, an example of a program involving this type of training is PROMPT (Sohlberg et al., 1985). The therapist asks the patient to remember to organize a target task within a specific number of minutes (for example, *I want you to open this envelope in 5 minutes*). The number of minutes is increased after the client demonstrates repeated success at a particular time interval. Throughout the training, the therapist systematically increases the time the client can remember and act on the assigned task.

Some variables should be selected according to the patient's current level of functioning:

- Type of task (motor command or functional task): *Example of motor command*: clapping hands; an *example of a functional task*: opening the envelope, sorting papers, "serving tea" to the dolls, putting the cars in the "garage".
- Increase of time (number of minutes between the administration and execution of the task).
- Distractor task during the interval.
- Associated stimuli to initiate the task (alarm or independent time control).

Prospective memory training is a specific restorative technique designed to increase the functioning of prospective memory with a satisfactory degree of generalization.

Expanded Rehearsal

The individual practices successful retrieval of information through gradually longer time intervals (Bjork, 1988). The longer the distractor interval from the first to the second successful retrieval attempt, the greater the likelihood of retrieval on the third attempt. The target information is then said, and the client is immediately asked, aiming at information retrieval. In subsequent attempts, the client is asked to retrieve the information after time intervals that can be doubled as the training progresses. The time intervals are interspersed with conversation or therapy activities. If the client gives a wrong answer, the professional provides the correct information, asks for immediate retrieval, and returns to the last time interval. Some characteristics:

- Learning should be effortless (i.e., without rehearsal for memorization).
- The information or procedure to be taught should be concrete.
- Errors should be limited; that is, they should be avoided as much as possible for the patient to make mistakes during the learning rehearsal.
- A part of the information should be taught at a time.
- The extension of the intervals does not have to be exact. *Example:* 2 s, 5 s, 4 s, 9 s, and so on).

Generally, this technique is useful for learning keywords, name-face associations, procedures for using external memory devices and learning the names of objects.

Use of Priming or the Method of "Appearing Signs" or Disappearing Signs"

The method of "disappearing signs" or "appearing signs" can be used to teach complex knowledge or behaviors that could be used in daily life. Firstly, the patient is provided with enough information to give a correct response. Then, parts of the information are gradually withdrawn or presented through learning attempts so that the patient gradually receives the signs. Learning continues until there are no more visible visual cues, then distractors (*for example,* therapy tasks such as stimulation or conversations with the patient) are included until the name has been remembered in similar contexts in the patient's daily life (Glisky et al., 1986). See Tables 8.2 and 8.3 for some examples.

Table 8.2 Example of "appearing signs"

Travessa Nestor de Castro alley, 231
(15 s of presentation)
T _, _ _ _
(10 s without customer response)
T R _, _ _ _
(10 s without customer response)
T R A _ _ _ _ _ _ _ _ _ _ _ _ _ _ _ _ _ _ _, _ _ _

Table 8.3 Example of "disappearing signs"

Travessa Nestor de Castro Alley, 231
T R A V E S S A N E S T O R D E C A S T R O, 2 3 1
(patient receives the complete information for 10 s)
T R A V E S S A N E S T O R D E C A S T R O, 2 3 _
(10 seconds for some response to be offered)
T R A V E S S A N E S T O R D E C A S T R O, 2 _ _

Errorless Learning

Severely amnesic individuals can acquire new information. However, the nature of this acquisition is different than for neurologically healthy individuals:

- Learning is slow and requires more repetition.
- Instructions must be systematic.
- Non-declarative learning will serve as the basis for acquisition.

Errorless learning is an instructional method that reduces errors in the acquisition phase. Studies indicate that for some individuals and certain types of tasks, eliminating the opportunity to make errors when starting to learn a task will increase learning. Therapists prevent clients from making errors by providing systematic guidance in the initial acquisition phase, different from the test and correction approach. Two methods:

(c) Provide the correct answer to the client until the therapist judges that the client can respond correctly without assistance.
(d) Model a particular step or procedure for the client and ask him to imitate it until he is able to do it without demonstration.

The goal is to prevent the child and teenager from practicing the wrong answers. So, during the initial learning phase of a routine, of specific information or during the practice of cognitive stimulation through exercises and games, it is necessary to model the behavior of the child and teenager so that the therapist first provides the example and demonstrates to the patient what should be done, then, therapist and child practice together until they achieve independent work. In this method, practice is the presumed path through which most people learn.

Final Considerations

Memory alterations and impairments, in general, impact the academic performance and achievement of children and teenagers and harm various other life contexts. However, the current research situation on the effectiveness of compensatory strategies, accommodation strategies and cognitive training is still incipient. It does not provide a basis for the action and control of memory dysfunctions in the child population, even though such alterations present as common diagnoses in children with neurological or psychiatric problems or even associated with learning difficulties. Research on the effectiveness of cognitive memory training performance is focused on working memory. A good part of the tasks used in training are tasks that require repetition of digits or visualization of blocks, which are not very ecological and present low potential for generalization, making the results of these investigations provide little proof of the effectiveness of cognitive training. However, strategies combined with an individual rehabilitation plan based on objectives and focused on the patient's problem are the most suitable interventions. The chapter summarized possible strategies for the stimulation and rehabilitation of memory based on clinical evidence and experience accumulated by the author.

References

Anderson, J. R. (2004). *Psicologia Cognitiva e suas implicações experimentais*. LTC.

Atkinson, R. C., & Shiffrin, R. M. (1968). Human memory: A proposed system and its control processes. In K. W. Spence & J. T. Spence (Eds.), *The psychology of learning and motivation* (pp. 89–195). Academic Press.

Baddeley, A. (2003). Working memory: Looking back and looking forward. *Nature Reviews Neuroscience, 4*, 829–839. https://doi.org/10.1038/nrn1201

Baddeley, A. (2004). *Your memory: A user's guide*. Firefly Books.

Baddeley, A. D., & Hitch, G. (1974). Working memory. In G. H. Bower (Ed.), *The psychology of learning and motivation: Advances in research and theory* (pp. 47–89). Academic Press.

Bjork, R. A. (1988). Retrieval practice and the maintenance of knowledge. In M. Guneberg, P. E. Morris, & R. N. Sykes (Eds.), *Practical aspects of memory: Current research and issues* (pp. 81–85). Wiley.

Cohen, M. (1997). *Children's memory scale: Professional manual*. Psychological Corporation.

Conners, F. A., Rosenquist, C. J., Arnett, L., Moore, M. S., & Hume, L. E. (2008). Improving memory span in children with down syndrome. *Journal of Intellectual Disabilitiy Research, 52*, 244–255. https://doi.org/10.1111/j.1365-2788.2007.01015.x

Dehn, M. J. (2008). *Working memory and academic learning: Assessment and intervention*. Wiley.

Engle, R. W., Tuholski, S. W., Laughlin, J. E., & Conway, A. R. A. (1999). Working memory, short term memory, and general fluid intelligence: A latent-variable approach. *Journal of Experimental Psychology: General, 128*, 309–331.

Gazzaniga, M. S., Ivry, R. B. & Mangun, G. R. (2006). *Neurociência Cognitiva—A Biologia da Mente* (2ªEd). Artmed.

Glisky, E. L., & Glisky, M. L. (2002). Learning and memory impairments. In P. J. Eslinger (Ed.), *Neuropsychological interventions: Clinical research and practices* (pp. 137–162). Guilford.

Glisky, E. L., Schacter, D. L., & Tulving, E. (1986). Learning and retention of computer related vocabularyin amnesic patients: Method of vanishing cues. *Journal of Clinical and Experimental Neuropsychology, 8*, 292–312.

Grady, C. (1999). Neuroimaging and activation of the frontal lobes. In B. L. Miller & J. L. Cummings (Eds.), *The human frontal lobes: Functions and disorders* (pp. 196–230). Guilford Press.

Johnson, E., Humphrey, M., Mellard, D., Woods, K., & Swanson, H. L. (2010). Cognitive processing deficits and students with specific learning disabilities: A selective meta-analysis of the literature. *Learning Disabilities, 33*(1), 3–18. https://doi.org/10.1177/073194871003300101

Martin, R. C. (2003). Language processing: Functional organization and neuroanatomical basis. *Annual Review of Psychology, 54*, 55–89.

Miller, D. C. (2007). *Essentials of school neuropsychology assessment*. Wiley.

Miller, J. A., & Blasik, J. L. (2010). Assessing and interventions with children with memory and learning disorders. In J. A. Miller (Ed.), *Best practices in school neuropsychology* (pp. 641–671). Wiley.

Muller, N. C. K., Konrad, B. N., Kohn, N., Muñoz-Lopez, M., Czisch, M., Gernández, G., & Dresler, M. (2018). Hippocampal-caudate nucleus interactions support exceptional memory performance. *Brain Structure Function, 223*(3), 1379–1389. https://doi.org/10.1007/s00429-017-1556-2

Pascoe, L., Roberts, G., Doyle, L. W., Lee, K. J., Thompson, D. K., Seal, M. L., Josev, E. K., Nosarti, C., Gathercole, S., & Anderson, P. J. (2013). Preventing academic difficulties in preterm children: A randomised controls trial of an adaptive working memory training intervention. *Pediatrics, 13*(144), 1471–2431. https://doi.org/10.1186/1471-2431-13-144

Postle, B. R. (2007). Activated long-term memory? The bases of representation in working memory. In N. Osaka, R. H. Logie, & M. D. Esposito (Eds.), *The cognitive neuroscience of working memory* (pp. 333–350). Oxford University Press.

Rode, C., Robson, R., Purviance, A., Geary, D. C., & Mayr, U. (2014). Is working memory training effective? A study in school setting. *PLos One, 9*(8).

Rourke, B. P. (1994). Neuropsychological assessment of children with learning disabilities: Measurement issues. In C. R. Lyon (Ed.), *Frames of reference for the assessment of learning disabilities: New views on measurement issues* (pp. 475–514). Paul H. Brookes.

Smith, C. N. (2014). Retrograde memory for public events in mild cognitive impairment and its relationship to anterograde memory and neuroanatomy. *Neuropsychology, 28*(6), 959–972. https://doi.org/10.1037/neu0000117

Sohlberg, M. M., & Mateer, C. A. (2011). *Reabilitação Cognitiva: Uma Abordagem Neuropsicológica*. Editora Santos.

Sohlberg, M. M., & Turkstra, L. S. (2011). *Optimizing cognitive rehabilitation: Effective instructional methods*. Guilford Press.

Sohlberg, M. M., Mateer, C. A., & Geyer, S. (1985). *Prospective memory process training (PROMPT)*. Lash & Associates.

Stuss, D., & Benson, F. (1986). *The frontal lobes*. Raven Press.

Tulving, E. (2002). Episodic memory: From mind to brain. *Annual Review of Psychology, 53*, 1–25.

Tulving, E., & Marcovitch, H. L. (1998). Episodic and declarative memory: The role of the hippocampus. *The Hip, 8*, 198–204.

Wilson, B. A. (1987). *Rehabilitation of memory*. Guilford Press.

Wilson, B. A. (2009). *Reabilitação da Memória: Integrando teoria e prática*. Artmed.

Work, P. H. L., & Choi, H. (2005). Developing classroom and group interventions based on a neuropsychology paradigma. In R. C. D'Amato, E. Fletcher-Janzen, & C. R. Reynolds (Eds.), *Handbook of school neuropsychology*. Wiley.

Chapter 9
Executive Functions: Rehabilitation and Promotion in Childhood

Natália Martins Dias, Caroline de Oliveira Cardoso, and Chrissie Ferreira de Carvalho

Executive Functions: Definition, Models, and Associated Difficulties

From an early age, children are asked to control their behavior and how they express their emotions; they need to think of alternatives to solve problems, for example, during a game, play, or in their interactions. Already in the early years of formal schooling, they are asked to work independently to complete projects; they must organize and plan to meet goals. In addition, academic or social success will depend on the ease with which they can organize, prioritize, memorize and manipulate information or inhibit inappropriate behavior. That is, it is essential that children can develop or improve these skills (Meltzer, 2014). Such skills are known in neuropsychology as executive functions (EF), which can be understood as an umbrella concept that involves a series of cognitive processes responsible for directing behavior, thought, and emotions (Diamond, 2013; Miyake et al., 2000; Stelzer et al., 2010).

Diamond (2013) composed a theoretical model based on literature that considers three basic core components: working memory, inhibitory control (including self-control and interference control), and cognitive flexibility. According to the model, the core functions lay the foundations for more complex and higher-level functions, such as planning, decision-making, and problem-solving.

N. M. Dias (✉) · C. F. de Carvalho
Universidade Federal de Santa Catarina, Florianópolis, Santa Catarina, Brazil
e-mail: natalia.m.dias@ufsc.br; chrissie.carvalho@ufsc.br

C. O. Cardoso
Universidade Feevale, Novo Hamburgo, Rio Grande do Sul, Brazil
e-mail: carolinecardoso@feevale.br

C. O. Cardoso, N. M. Dias (eds.), *Neuropsychological Interventions for Children - Volume 1*, https://doi.org/10.1007/978-3-031-53586-4_9

The development of EF begins in childhood and continues until the end of adolescence and the beginning of adulthood (Center on the Developing Child at Harvard University, 2011; Hughes, 2011). However, the executive components do not mature at the same time, and their progression is mainly related to the maturation of the structures in the prefrontal region (Best & Miller, 2010; Rothlisberger et al., 2012). Inhibitory control, for example, begins its development earlier, followed by working memory and flexibility, which seem to develop later, with continuous development throughout adolescence (Best & Miller, 2010; Wu et al., 2011).

In addition to biological aspects, environment and social factors also influence the development of EF. Among the social factors, the socioeconomic level and parents' education stand out (Engel de Abreu et al., 2014a; Evans & Fuller-Rowell, 2013; Farah et al., 2006). Considering socioeconomic level, studies reveal that children from lower socioeconomic levels perform worse on tests that assess EF (Hackman et al., 2015). One study found that public school children performed worse than private school children in tasks measuring attention, planning, inhibition, and cognitive flexibility (Shayer et al., 2015). Other studies showed that children at socioeconomic disadvantage and poverty performed worse, mainly in components involving executive control and language (Farah et al., 2006; Lipina et al., 2013).

Academic performance is another factor correlated with EF ability, and individual differences in early childhood have been indicated as predictors of academic performance in later years (Blair & Razza, 2007; Ribner et al., 2017). A recent study evaluated 552 preschool children, and the results indicated that performance in EF tasks at 2 years old predicted emerging math and language skills at 5 years old, with this prediction being stronger for the area of math (Mulder et al., 2017). Indeed, the literature has highlighted the importance of EF for performance in math (Hornung et al., 2014; Van der Ven et al., 2012) and reading (Engel de Abreu et al., 2014b).

Given their importance for various outcomes throughout life, such as academic performance (Bierman et al., 2008; Blair & Diamond, 2008) and professional success (Prince et al., 2007), children with deficits in these skills may experience many short and long-term impairments. Table 9.1 presents examples of difficulties that children with impairment in a certain component may manifest at home, at school, and when establishing interpersonal relationships.

Thus, given the relevance of EF for various areas throughout life, as well as the social, emotional, academic and professional consequences that dysfunction can cause, there is increasingly more investment in neuropsychological interventions aimed at rehabilitating or enhancing these skills, even at stages of the life cycle where these skills are still in development. Promoting EF can have a direct and long-term impact on academic performance, reduce school lag, and prevent social and mental health problems, such as addiction to psychoactive substances and behavioral issues (Roebers et al., 2011; Zito et al., 2000).

Table 9.1 Executive functions and difficulties in different contexts

	Examples of difficulty in different contexts/situations		
Ability	School	Home	Social relations
Inhibition	Does not pay attention in class (difficulty in attention control) Has impulsive responses Difficulties in controlling their behavior Gets distracted easily and has difficulty maintaining focus	Interrupts adult conversations Interrupts parents when they are speaking, speaks out of turn Difficulty following routines and rules, which requires persistence for their implementation	Acts impulsively, says what they should not or behaves without considering others May have difficulties keeping secrets May be seen as "annoying" or a friend who bothers, as they disturb others and may have difficulty dealing with frustration
Working memory	Does not follow/ remember instructions to the end Difficulties in understanding what they read and doing mental calculations May have disorganized writing and speech	Gets lost in the middle of activities Tends not to finish tasks Difficulty following instructions with many steps	Is late or simply forgets commitments Difficulty following a long conversation or one with many pieces of information
Flexibility	Difficulty switching or changing from one activity to another Difficulty understanding figurative information Even when making a mistake, cannot change the way they perform an activity	Thinking tends to be rigid and concrete Does not show "creativity" in trying to solve problems (making a recipe when missing an ingredient, for example)	Difficulty understanding others' points of view Wants things to always be done their way May have difficulty understanding jokes and irony/ sarcasm
Organization and planning	Misses deadlines and due dates for assignments May have several ideas and be creative, but when starting the activity does not know how to organize project stages	Their study area and/or room is disorganized Does not plan or gets lost even when performing household tasks	Can be seen as careless or irresponsible Colleagues may avoid him for schoolwork or other situations
Emotion regulation	Easily frustrated in the face of difficulties May overreact to certain situations May have difficulty expressing his emotions appropriately, with consequences for his relationships with peers May have difficulty controlling emotions such as anger and sadness, possibly acting aggressively or impulsively		

Re(h)abilitation of Executive Functions in Childhood

The intervention on EF aims to achieve the best possible adaptation of the individual in his daily life, enabling a better quality of life from stimulating cognitive processes that allow the control and regulation of behavior. There is increasing evidence suggesting that EF can be improved through training and stimulation (Cardoso et al., 2016, Diamond & Lee, 2011).

Dawson and Guare (2014) propose three general strategies to stimulate EF in children and adolescents: (1) Intervene in the environment, (2) Teach skills, and (3) Motivate the child to use executive skills. Such strategies are not exclusive and can be used mutually throughout rehabilitation.

1. Intervene in the environment—It consists of identifying ways to modify the environment surrounding the child. It also includes changing the task or the way people (parents and teachers) interact with the child. For example, modifying the environment includes reducing distractors, such as placing the child with attention difficulties closer to the teacher and away from the window, using organizational structures (folders, labels, colors). Task modifications may mean shortening tasks, creating breaks or making tasks more explicit. Finally, changing the form of interaction includes providing more frequent cues and reminders, verbally reinforcing the child when they manage to perform the requested task (for example, *I liked the way you organized your room*).
2. Teach executive skills—It consists of teaching the target skill. That is, providing direct and explicit instructions about the strategy to be perfected or developed. Cognitive training aimed at stimulating the executive skill desired can be included. First, the problem behavior and goals are defined, then strategies are developed and implemented to minimize the problem behavior or enhance the skill. In the initial stage, the child will need to be instructed on how to achieve the goal and be supervised, with the monitoring gradually decreasing and the child becoming more independent.
3. Motivate the child to use executive skills—An efficient strategy is to positively reinforce the change, which motivates the child to modify their behavior. For example, for a child who resists doing household chores, adults can combine a pleasurable activity after its completion (such as being able to watch a show or play for 15 min). Other examples that can motivate the child to use the skill would be to alternate between preferred and non-preferred activity, provide breaks or use praise to reinforce a certain behavior.

In rehabilitation and habilitation, there are well-established proposals in the literature that, although outlined for adults, are also used for teenagers or even adapted for children. Among these proposals, and in line with the idea also presented by Dawson and Guare (2014), is the intervention for EF by Sohlberg and Mateer (2001). The authors suggest strategies, such as:

(a) Environmental control (i.e., providing an organization of the environment to reduce the demand on the EF, e.g., use of a calendar for planning, external devices _ like cell phone alarm _ to assist with reminders);
(b) Specific routines for tasks (i.e., a routine is created for a specific activity and training is promoted aiming at its automation, minimizing the executive demand);
(c) Training in the selection and execution of plans (provide practice in planning and executing tasks, exercising executive skills in hypothetical activities or real situations); and
(d) Metacognitive strategies/self-instructional training (teach the patient to use strategies to support the regulation of their behavior; this includes strategies such as verbal self-instruction and well-established techniques like the *Goal management training* _ GMT).

A type of strategy widely used, especially in rehabilitation, is cognitive training. Various resources are available, from board games and pencil and paper activities to computerized training (Diamond & Lee, 2011). Regarding computerized training, working memory is the skill that has been the focus of investment. In a summary description, these are exercises developed based on (or similar to) testing paradigms. They offer the opportunity for repeated practice in adaptive activities, or with a graded level of difficulty, adjusted according to the individual's performance. Working memory training has been used both in the context of rehabilitation, as in children with traumatic brain injury (Phillips et al., 2016), as well as habilitation, as is the case of the study by Bennett et al. (2013) with children with Down Syndrome, as well as in children with learning disorders, which usually have deficits in working memory (Peijnenborgh et al., 2016). Despite some evidence like the references mentioned above, it is worth noting that many criticisms have been addressed to computerized training, especially regarding the non-transfer of gains to untrained skills and for functioning in the "real world" (Sala et al., 2018).

A criticism of cognitive training suggests that providing a game environment or practice in computerized programs alone may not sufficiently stimulate EF. Children must understand their cognitive profile and be taught to observe, evaluate, monitor, and manage their executive skills (Cardoso et al., 2016; Riccio & Gomes, 2013). Through psychoeducation, professionals present strengths and weaknesses, teaching which strategies work well for the child and why, where, when, and how to use specific strategies. Knowledge about their cognitive processes and strategies, known as metacognition, allows the child to better understand their abilities, increasing their self-efficacy and self-confidence (Meltzer, 2010, 2014). Adults (parents, teachers, and therapists) play a crucial role in this process by initially showing and explaining what and how to do it, then verbally guiding and supervising until the child can perform the task independently. Adults need to provide opportunities for children to develop their executive functions (EF) (Cardoso & Holmer, 2018).

Considering metacognitive strategies, GMT, mentioned earlier, is a training to teach the patient to "stop" an automatic behavior and set goals or steps in conducting an activity. A recent study applied GMT to adolescents between 11 and 17 years old with complaints of difficulties in EF inside and outside the school context. The intervention was conducted in 8 sessions, and the contents included the concept of "autopilot," "STOP" strategies (focus on stopping automatic behaviors), checking the "Mental Blackboard" (access and training of working memory), setting goals, decision making and breaking down complex tasks into smaller steps. There is also encouragement to monitor performance. The group participating in the intervention had gains mainly in inhibition and flexibility, as well as in general intelligence and working memory, the latter observed during performance in an ecological task. Follow-up analysis (4 weeks) also showed problem-solving and planning gains (Nunes, 2017).

Another very structured proposal is brought by Meltzer (2010), addressed to elementary and high school students with or without attentional and/or learning difficulties (it can also be used in the context of habilitation or early-preventive/promotion). Meltzer's (2010) proposal emphasizes the explicit and systematic teaching of strategies that involve skills of goal setting, planning and prioritization, organization, working memory, flexibility and self-monitoring, in addition to emotional self-regulation. Many strategies are used in the context of school content areas, such as reading and math. Here is a summary of some of his suggestions:

- *Goal setting*: Use of calendar or timeline; provide students with an understanding of the "whole," the final goal of the task and, subsequently, help them to establish sub-goals;
- *Planning and prioritization*: Teach children to categorize their activities (obligations, fun, other activities) and set up individualized daily schedules for organizing their daily routine;
- *Organization*: Encourage periodic checking of the study environment, folders or backpack (which can be done with the help of a *checklist*). In idea organization, aid strategies can be used, for example, in writing or reading texts. The STAR strategy is suggested, in which students use the drawing of a star as a graphic organizer. Thus, at each point of the star, they write a question to be addressed in their narrative (writing planning) to organize information such as: Who, Where, How, When and Why.
- *Memory*: Encourage the use of strategies such as: (1) paying attention to details (includes the use of visual resources, like different colors); (2) repetition, rehearsal and review (e.g. rehearsing the information out loud, writing it and reading it); (3) assigning meaning (can use maps or diagrams to organize the information and create associations with what they already know about a topic); and (4) aggregating information (combining items, composing a smaller number of data units). The use of acronyms is also suggested (about this, see Chap. 8).
- *Flexibility*: Activities that give students the opportunity to solve problems from different perspectives; activities in pairs or groups, where they need to deal with different points of view.
- *Self-monitoring:* Clearly communicate your expectations to the student. Encourage the review of work and try to identify your most common mistakes, which can lead to creating a *checklist* for verification.

- *Emotional regulation:* The professional should provide a model (express their emotions and appropriate ways to manage them); he/she should model and teach self-instructions that help deal with stressful situations. Activities of *role-play* allow for the simulation of emotional regulation in different contexts. Discussion about inappropriate behaviors and their impact on others is encouraged.

Promotion of Executive Functions in Childhood—Preventive Interventions

In 2007, Diamond et al. (2007) pointed out that most EF interventions designed for children aimed to remedy deficits rather than promote such skills or prevent difficulties. More than a decade later, we can affirm that there has been progress in relation to that scenario. Over the past few years, we have seen the development and study of programs and other initiatives aimed at stimulating EF with a focus on promoting these skills in non-clinical contexts.

Regarding different approaches used in EF stimulation, according to Diamond and Lee (2011) one can consider:

- *Computerized training*: This approach to rehabilitation has already been presented in our previous topic but has also been employed in healthy/typical populations for promotion purposes. A relevant aspect is that such tools focus on specific skills. Evidence summarized by Diamond and Lee (2011) suggests that computerized training can promote gains in the trained task without evidence of generalization for untrained skills.
- *Computerized and non-computerized games*: This approach considers using games in different formats. There is some evidence of the effectiveness of these tools, including gains in school performance, although this seems specific to the participants with the greatest delay (Goldin et al., 2014). In Brazil, research groups have dedicated themselves to developing and studying games as cognitive promotion tools; it is pertinent to share a little of this experience worldwide. Among these initiatives, one can mention the studies with the School of the Brain, whose use of cognitive games has been shown to be associated with improvement in attention measures, in addition to teachers' reports about maintaining attention for a longer time in activities, faster problem-solving, and even improvement in children's social skills (Ramos, 2015). Another important initiative in the area is from the Virtual Communities group at UNEB, which contributes to the insertion of games in learning spaces (Torres & Alves, 2013). The group developed the *Gamebook* Guardians of the Forest, an *appbook* that integrates book narrative with games in an interactive environment (Guimarães et al. 2016). More information about the role of games and digital technologies in neuropsychological intervention can be consulted in Chap. 9 of the second volume of *Neuropsychological Interventions for Children*. In the same book, Chap. 12 also discusses the use of games and play for intervention.

- *Aerobic exercises*: Diamond and Lee (2011) summarize some studies that suggest EF gains in children from 8 to 12 years of age with aerobic exercises. They point out, however, that greater gain seems to be related to the greater demand of the activity on the executive skills and postulate that regular sports practice can impact EF even more than aerobic activities. One of the reasons would be linked to the fact that sports, especially team ones, demand executive skills, such as sustained attention, working memory, and discipline, in addition to promoting group interaction.
- *Martial arts and mental contemplation practices* (*mindfulness*): The development of self-control and discipline are among the focuses of practices such as martial arts, with evidence that children who practice regularly have greater gains in EF. Mindfulness practices contribute to the development of attention control and self-monitoring, with evidence of generalization of gains to other areas and activities (Diamond & Lee, 2011). For example, Flook et al. (2010) showed evidence of gains in behavior regulation, metacognition, and overall executive control of children aged 7–9 who started the study with poorer EF after 8 weeks of participation in a *mindfulness* program, suggesting that the practice can be especially important for children with executive difficulties. Further information about Mindfulness can be found in Chap. 10 of Volume 2 of *Neuropsychological Interventions for Children.*
- *School curriculums*: Perhaps the most studied curriculum promoting EF is the Tools of the Mind, a preschool curriculum focused on developing skills relevant to the literacy stage. In addition to the initial studies in this area that tested the *Tools* (e.g. Barnett et al., 2008; Diamond et al., 2007), more recent evidence suggests that intervention with the *Tools* can minimize the *gap* in school performance between children from poorer homes compared to their peers from higher-income families. The authors found that, in addition to greater gains in measures of EF, the children (5 years old) who participated in the *Tools* had greater gains in reasoning and math and, in *follow-up* 1 year after the end of the intervention, they still had better performance in vocabulary, reading, and math. Some of these gains, however, were specific to the poorest schools. Also, an effect of the intervention on the salivary cortisol level was found, suggesting an impact on the stress regulation system (Blair & Raver, 2014). In addition to the *Tools*, Diamond and Lee (2011) also mention the Montessori curriculum for its encouragement of self-discipline and independence.
- *Complementary curricular programs*: These offer a structure and specific strategies to be implemented in conjunction with the regular curriculum. An example mentioned by Diamond and Lee (2011) is PATH (*Promoting Alternative Thinking Strategies*). The focus is on the development of self-control, recognition and management of feelings and resolution of interpersonal problems in children through their teachers' training and application of the program.

Beyond the approaches presented by Diamond and Lee (2011), other authors have included brief curricular programs with the participation of parents. For example, the program "*Ready? Set. Go!*" (RSG) was designed to promote EF in preschoolers in vulnerable situations, such as homeless children or those with high housing instability

(Casey et al., 2014). The program has three components: (1) teacher training and classroom curriculum: introduction about the concepts and importance of EF for academic success, encouragement to teachers to bring their own ideas for the promotion of EF and the presentation of the program's activities; (2) Parent Training and Involvement: Sessions with parents that involve both psychoeducational aspects and interaction with the child through music and games that will stimulate EF and generate moments of positive interaction between parents and children, in addition to sending explanatory materials and games home; (3) Child training and individual level support: through the indication of greater needs for EF intervention. The RSG was developed based on the theory of Change with a focus on EF and, according to the authors (Casey et al., 2014), needs further studies to improve its benefits.

Evidence-Based Programs Available in the Brazilian Context: Sharing Our Practice with the World

The programs highlighted below represent Brazilian initiatives. They start from a common principle: to provide means and opportunities for practice and, consequently, for the development of EF, preparing children to deal with the increasing demands of school and society. It is worth noting that this panorama is not exhaustive, with other equally relevant interventions being developed in various countries. Let's explore some of these programs that have made a difference in Brazil.

The *Glia Method* (Arruda & Mata, 2014a, b; Arruda et al., 2015) is a program based on two stages: evaluation and intervention. In the evaluation stage, from scales filled out by parents, teachers and the individual himself, it is possible to outline the areas of greatest difficulty and need for intervention. In turn, the intervention stage is designed for clinical, school and family contexts. The intervention targets are: Mental health, resilience, social skills, EF (cold and hot[1]), metacognition and school motivation. It is aimed at children and adolescents from 6 to 18 years old with or without behavior, emotional and learning problems and is operationalized from three books, which bring the strategies and structure of the intervention work: the *parents' book*, which provides information about EF and its development, gives clues on how parents can identify difficulties in these skills and presents tips on strategies for EF to be stimulated in a family context; the *teachers' book* presents a program divided into two stages: 11 weeks focusing on the development of EF and 6 weeks for work with metacognition, from daily activities (30 min). Each EF and each metacognitive strategy is worked on for 1 week, covering from the presentation of each skill to its exercise in practical activities. *The therapist's book* brings the technical principles of the intervention, which guide the sessions for work with each skill (around seven sessions for each EF).

[1] Cold EF: Cognitive aspect of executive functions. Skills implicated in situations with minimal demands on emotional/motivational processes. Hot EF: Top-down *control* exercised in situations with significant emotional or motivational load; includes emotional regulation, social behaviors, and decision-making.

The Neuropsychological Rehabilitation Program for Executive Functions in Students with Developmental Dyslexia (PRN-D from the name in Portuguese *Programa de Reabilitação Neuropsicológica para as funções executivas em estudantes com Dislexia do desenvolvimento*) was developed and tested by Lima (2015) and is a specific program aimed at stimulating EF in students with dyslexia. The program stimulates self-regulated learning, study skills (such as organization of environment and materials, note-taking, homework, and use of time), and reading competence. The PRN-D develops over 30 sessions, one to two times a week, conducted individually, and is structured in four modules: Psychoeducation, Orientation, Executive functions applied to study skills, and Executive Functions applied to reading comprehension. The efficacy study of the program revealed improvements in the performance of the experimental group, formed by six students (aged between 12 and 15 years) with dyslexia, in measures of EF, in addition to gains in the use of learning and comprehension strategies, and in reading comprehension itself. There were also reports of gains in performance in attention and processing speed and a decrease in teacher complaints about difficulties in EF. A single case analysis (boy, 13 years old, diagnosed with dyslexia) also revealed gains in EF, repertoire of learning strategies and comprehension, and reading comprehension (Lima, 2015).

Furthermore, in terms of rehabilitation and habilitation of EF, it is worth mentioning Brazilian initiatives that include the development of interactive media, such as a *gamebook* for stimulating EF in children and adolescents with Attention Deficit Hyperactivity Disorder (ADHD) (Rocha et al., 2014). Also in the scope of habilitation, two adaptations of the Intervention Program in Self-Regulation and Executive Functions (PIAFEx; presented later in this chapter) were carried out: One is for adolescents with ADHD, which was tested in a clinical context, in group therapy, with promising results (Menezes et al., 2015). The other is the adaptation of activities for work with children and adolescents with Down Syndrome (Freire, 2018). The Mind Heroes program, also presented in this chapter, is in the process of adaptation to the clinical context and is being tested in children with ADHD.

Evidence-Based Promotion Programs Available in Brazil

The following programs were developed for (primary) use in the school context, applied by the teachers themselves and with a preventive character.

1. ***Intervention Program in Self-Regulation and Executive Functions—PIAFEx (from the name in Portuguese 'Programa de Intervenção em Autorregulação e Funções Executivas')***

   PIAFEx (Dias & Seabra, 2013) was published in 2013; it is the pioneer program in Brazil focusing on promoting EF in children in Early Childhood Education and first grade of Elementary School. It is divided into a section of *Essential Aspects*, which includes tips on strategies and ways of interaction for promoting EF, ten basic modules and one complementary. The modules are presented in Table 9.2.

Table 9.2 Modules of PIAFEx

Module 1—Organization of Materials/Routine and Time Management	Strategies aimed at assisting organization and time management during classroom activities
Module 2—Organization of ideas, establishment of goals and plans: Daily strategies	Strategies to assist in organization and planning for project execution and goal setting
Module 3—Organization of ideas, establishment of goals and plans: Stimulation activities	Activities that demand executive skills, including organization of ideas and understanding of the consequences of behavior
Module 4—Executive functions in physical/motor activities	Activities that mainly involve inhibition and attention in the context of games and play
Module 5—Communication and conflict management	Strategies/activities to provide children with the opportunity to learn behavior and emotion regulation strategies, aiming to teach appropriate means of resolving interpersonal conflicts
Module 6—Regulating emotions	Activities to teach children to recognize and deal with their emotions, including modeling and practicing appropriate ways of expressing them
Module 7—Working with peers—The *opportunity to exercise hetero and self-regulation*	Activities that require interaction and cooperation, where children have different roles but share a common goal. It involves hetero and self-regulation of behavior
Module 8—Playing with the meanings of words	Activities to stimulate thought flexibility
Module 9—Talking about activities	Stimulates reflection on one's own strategies and thought processes
Module 10—The planned play	A pretend-play game structured in three stages: Planning, execution, and evaluation. The activity allows for the stimulation of working memory, flexibility, and inhibitory control, in addition to practicing such skills (and others, such as creativity, vocabulary, problem-solving, social skills, etc.) in various play contexts
Complementary module: Nina's diary	A narrative that introduces the character Nina and her friends. The characters encounter situations and need to learn ways to deal with them, serving as a model and presenting strategies for emotion regulation, planning, and organization, among others. There are suggested activities for practice after each chapter

Evidence of PIAFEx Effectiveness Compared to the regular school curriculum, greater gains in attention and inhibition were observed in preschool children who participated in the intervention with PIAFEx (Dias & Seabra, 2015a). In first-grade classes, gains were observed in attention, inhibition, flexibility, and planning (Dias & Seabra, 2015b). More recently, a study found a transfer of gains to reading, math, and behavior measures (such as a lower rate of peer problems and a higher rate of pro-social behavior), with the maintenance of gains even 1 year after the end of the intervention (Dias & Seabra, 2017).

2. ***Neuropsychological Stimulation Program of Cognition in Students—Emphasis on Executive Functions—PENcE (from the name in Portuguese 'Programa de Estimulação Neuropsicológica da Cognição em Escolares: Ênfase nas Funções Executivas')***
   The PENcE (Cardoso & Fonseca, 2016) is an intervention aimed at stimulating and enhancing executive skills and was developed for school-aged children, specifically for Elementary School I. Through a narrative of a story and various playful and cognitive activities, children are encouraged to think about their own cognitive processes and appropriate the taught strategies so that they can, from then on, use them in other everyday situations and other school subjects. The program was organized into four modules and each module is made up of three stages, as can be seen in Table 9.3.

Table 9.3 Organization of the PENcE program

Modules	Organization of the modules and activities
Module 1—Planning and organization	Stage 1: Strategy acquisition—psychoeducation and modeling—represented by Beatriz the Ant Stage 2: Learning and consolidation of the strategy—Activities = fitting the numbers; dot game; in search of the diamond; logical sequence; building an insect; cooking Stage 3: Reflections and transfer to everyday life—space for exchanges and reflections on how to use the strategies in other situations beyond school
Module 2—Inhibitory control	Stage 1: Strategy acquisition—psychoeducation and modeling—represented by Pedro the Ant Stage 2: Learning and consolidation of the strategy—Activities = dancing; searching for the target; controlling the desire; Simon says; card game bate-bate; each sound, a movement Stage 3: Reflections and transfer to everyday life—space for exchanges and reflections on how to use the strategies in other situations beyond school
Module 3—Working memory	Stage 1: Strategy acquisition—psychoeducation and modeling—represented by Patricia the Ant Stage 2: Learning and consolidation of the strategy—Activities = organizing the sequences; difference game; missing 1; completing the sentence; numbering the sequence. Stage 3: Reflections and transfer to everyday life—space for exchanges and reflections on how to use the strategies in other situations beyond school
Module 4—Cognitive flexibility	Stage 1: Strategy acquisition—psychoeducation and modeling—Represented by Fabio the Ant Stage 2: Learning and consolidation of the strategy—Activities = looking from another perspective; swap-swap; matching the cards; discover the code; A new ending Stage 3: Reflections and transfer to everyday life—space for exchanges and reflections on how to use the strategies in other situations beyond school

Evidence of PENcE Effectiveness The children who participated in PENcE showed significant gains in inhibitory control, working memory and planning compared to children who remained with the regular curriculum. In addition, there was a transfer effect to other cognitive skills (attention, initiation, processing speed, short-term memory, fluid reasoning), academic skills (mathematics and word writing) and behavior change (higher mental health index, lower index of relationship and conduct problems) (Cardoso, 2017).

3. ***Executive Functions Stimulation Program—Mind Heroes***

   The Mind Heroes Program (MHP) was developed to work playfully the concepts of EF in children between 7 and 12 years old in a school context and also has a version for a clinical context (Carvalho, 2017; Carvalho & Abreu, 2023). The program revolves around the story of the Mind Heroes, three characters who acquired their hero skills because they have difficulties in EF and, because of this, they help other children with problems in planning, organization, working memory, inhibitory control and emotional regulation. The content of the MHP consists of six comic stories that are the basis for the proposed activities, which are divided into four modules presented in Table 9.4.

Table 9.4 Modules of the Mind Heroes program

Integrating module	
Comic Story—Mind Heroes: 6 stories It focuses on the Metacognition skill, which permeates the entire program. The stories generate content and models for the modules.	
Module 1 *Organization and Planning* 11 activities Daily routine. Learning to make plans. Use of the calendar. Time management. Organization of physical space and ideas in texts and stories. Organization of sequences. Logic tasks.	*Module 2* *Attention, Inhibitory Control and Cognitive Flexibility* 17 activities Stop and think before acting. Games and activities that require inhibitory control. Cognitive flexibility tasks: spelling, problem-solving, stories with multiple endings, and mimicry. Exploring ambiguous sentences. Activities of categorizing words and images.
Module 3 *Working and prospective memory* 7 activities Learning to make a checklist. Adding rules and retaining new information in games and play. Recalling activities with calendar support. Immediate memory game and with interference.	*Module 4* *Emotions and self-regulation* 6 activities Identification and expression of emotions (drawing, imitating). Everyday situations and identification of the emotions generated. Teaching and monitoring the use of strategies for emotional regulation and behavior. Empathy and self-regulation.

Evidence of PHM Effectiveness The results of the efficacy study indicated benefits achieved by children who participated in the PHM from public schools in the metropolitan region of Salvador (Carvalho, 2017). When compared to the control group, the group of children exposed to manganese, considered more vulnerable, showed gains in measures of working memory, cognitive flexibility, phonemic verbal fluency, visual and auditory-verbal attention and transfer to writing, while the group without a history of exposure showed gains related to processing speed in tasks of inhibitory control, cognitive flexibility, and decision-making. The control group was the only one that showed a reduction in scores in Fluid Intelligence. It was demonstrated that the PHM had a protective effect on fluid intelligence and children in a situation of greater vulnerability benefited more from the PHM for the promotion of EF.

4. ***Training of Educators on Neuropsychology of Learning: Emphasis on Executive Functions and Attention—CENA***

   The CENA (Pureza & Fonseca, 2016) consists of a training program for elementary school educators to provide teachers with greater knowledge about EF so that they can develop strategies to stimulate these skills in their students. The intervention was developed to be carried out in 11 meetings. The initial meeting aims to address the basic notions about neuropsychology and its applicability to the field of education. The intermediate sessions are structured from the main components of EF and related processes applied to education. At this point, some guidelines, tips, and activities are provided to teachers. To conclude, the last session provides the opportunity to perform exercises for assimilation and understanding of the contents worked on during the intervention.

Tips for Stimulation (Habilitation, Rehabilitation, or Promotion) of Executive Functions

Table 9.5 presents tips for strategies and tasks to stimulate each component of the EF in various age groups, whether with a focus on promotion or rehabilitation.

Final Considerations

EF is a fundamental skill for school performance and the individual's social functioning. Therefore, talking about stimulating these skills is so relevant in the clinical or educational context. The chapter summarized existing models and presented some of the initiatives and tools we have developed in Brazil for the international audience. Despite this, some gaps are still obvious, such as structured programs developed for implementation in high school. However, adapting activities from

Table 9.5 Tips for stimulating EF in various age groups

Skills/strategies/tips	Adolescence		Childhood	
	ECE	EE I	EE II	HS
Inhibitory control				
Games that stimulate behavior inhibition and attention: Statue, dead-alive, hit right, etc.	x	x		
Activities in which they must inhibit automatic behavior, for example, during a presentation, do not say certain words		x	x	x
Strategy: Self-instruction—teach to use "internal speech" before any activity: "STOP" and think before proceeding	x	x	x	x
Environment modification: remove distractors, take more frequent breaks	x	x	x	x
Working memory				
Games in which the child must keep information in mind, like "telephone game," but with sentences or more than one word (progressively increase the number of words)	x	x		
Organize sequences of figures and create a narrative	x	x		
Exercises with mental calculations		x	x	x
Strategy: when it is necessary to do more than one activity at the same time or when there is a lot of information, encourage them to pay attention, memorize, and then organize and manipulate the stimuli mentally		x	x	x
Environment modification: provide clear and objective instructions without too much information at the same time	x	x	x	x
Flexibility				
"Brainstorm" game—encourage coming up with different solutions for everyday problems		x	x	x
Encourage thinking about the meaning of popular sayings	x	x		
Strategy: In the face of a situation that needs to solve a problem, encourage them to think of different alternatives	x	x	x	x
Environment modification: promote changes that make routines and programs less rigid and more flexible	x	x	x	x
Organization and planning				
Games (Rush Hour, Peg Solitaire, UNO) in which you need to plan before executing to perform well	x	x	x	x
Plan a real activity: a family outing, packing a backpack, a recipe, building a game, etc.	x	x	x	
Strategy: encourage them to first plan, then execute, and finally, evaluate if what they planned was achieved	x	x	x	x
Strategy: encourage breaking down more complex activities into more manageable steps or stages	x	x	x	x
Strategy: stimulate prioritizing tasks by their urgency (deadline) and difficulty			x	x

(continued)

Table 9.5 (continued)

Skills/strategies/tips	Adolescence		Childhood	
	ECE	EE I	EE II	HS
Environment modification: use organizers to delineate the stages; use a calendar (collective for the little ones; individual for the older ones) or agenda and encourage daily review and anticipation of events	x	x	x	x
Emotion regulation				
Games or activities where the child needs to identify the emotions and relate them to situations already experienced. Activity in which they need to identify what happens in the body and face when they have a certain emotion	x	x		
Strategy: In situations of emotional excitement, validate and stimulate the child to identify what they are feeling	x	x		
Strategy: Use strategies that delay the response, such as "counting to 10" or breathing techniques	x	x	x	x
Strategy: Discuss inappropriate reactions and stimulate participants to come up with ways to regulate and deal with various situations	x	x	x	x
Environment modification: When the child presents some unpleasant emotion, validate it by asking them to express their feelings. Avoid punishing them or disqualifying what they are feeling	x	x	x	x

ECE—Early Childhood Education/EE—Elementary Education/HS—High School

existing programs and using strategies from internationally consolidated programs allow for meeting this demand. The authors hope that the summary provided here can guide the professionals in their search for models, programs and/or activities, stimulating the use, whether in rehabilitation, habilitation or promotion, of evidence-based practices.

References

Arruda, M. A., & Mata, M. F. (2014a). *Projeto Escola da Diversidade: Cartilha do Professor*. Ed. Instituto Glia.

Arruda, M. A., & Mata, M. F. (2014b). *Projeto Escola da Diversidade: Cartilha dos Pais e do Professor*. Ed. Instituto Glia.

Arruda, M. A., Pinheiro, C. Q., Barros, C., Mata, M. F., Rezende, G., & Arroyo, L. H. (2015). *Cartilha do Terapeuta. Método Glia*. Ed. Instituto Glia.

Barnett, W. S., Jung, K., Yarosz, D. J., Thomas, J., Hornbeck, A., Stechuk, R., & Burns, S. (2008). Early childhood research quarterly educational effects of the tools of the mind curriculum: A randomized trial. *Early Childhood Research Quarterly, 23*, 299–313. https://doi.org/10.1016/j.ecresq.2008.03.001

Bennett, S. J., Holmes, J., & Buckley, S. (2013). Computerized memory training leads to sustained improvement in visuospatial short-term memory skills in children with down syndrome. *American Journal on Intellectual and Developmental Disabilities, 118*(3), 179–192. https://doi.org/10.1352/1944-7558-118.3.179

Best, J. R., & Miller, P. H. (2010). A developmental perspective on executive function. *Child Development, 81*, 1641–1660.

Bierman, K. L., Nix, R. L., Greenberg, M. T., Blair, C., & Domitrovich, C. E. (2008). Executive functions and school readiness intervention: Impact, moderation, and mediation in the head start REDI program. *Development and Psychopathology, 20*, 821–843.

Blair, C., & Diamond, A. (2008). Biological processes in prevention and intervention: The promotion of self-regulation as a means of preventing school failure. *Development and Psychopathology, 20*, 899–891.

Blair, C., & Raver, C. C. (2014). Closing the achievement gap through modification of neurocognitive and neuroendocrine function: Results from a cluster randomized controlled trial of an innovative approach to the education of children in kindergarten. *PLoS One, 9*(11). https://doi.org/10.1371/journal.pone.0112393

Blair, C., & Razza, R. P. (2007). Relating effortful control, executive function, and false belief understanding to emerging math and literacy ability in kindergarten. *Child Development, 78*(2), 647–663. https://doi.org/10.1111/j.1467-8624.2007.01019.x

Cardoso, C. O. (2017). *Programas de intervenção neuropsicológica precoce-preventiva: estimulação das funções executivas em escolares (Tese de doutorado)*. Pontifícia Universidade Católica do Rio Grande do Sul.

Cardoso, C. O., & Fonseca, R. P. (2016). *Programa de Estimulação Neuropsicológica da Cognição em Escolares: ênfase nas Funções Executivas*. BookToy.

Cardoso, C. O., & Holmer, L. (2018). Responsabilidades: orientações sobre funções executivas. In D. Fava, M. Rosa, & A. D. Oliva (Eds.), *Orientação para pais—o que é preciso saber para cuidar dos filhos* (pp. 151–168). Artesã Editora.

Cardoso, C. O., Dias, N. M., Senger, J., Colling, A. P. C., Seabra, A. G., & Fonseca, R. P. (2016). Neuropsychological stimulation of executive functions in children with typical development: A systematic review. *Applied Neuropsychology: Child, 7*(1), 61–81. https://doi.org/10.1080/21622965.2016.1241950

Carvalho, C. F. (2017). *Programa de estimulação das funções executivas: contribuições para o desenvolvimento cognitivo de crianças em situação de vulnerabilidade e expostas ao manganês (Tese de Doutorado)*. Programa de Pós-graduação em Psicologia, Universidade Federal da Bahia.

Carvalho, C. F., & Abreu, N. (2023). *Heróis da Mente: caderno do aluno* (1st ed.). Ampla.

Casey, E. C., Finsaas, M., Carlson, S. M., Zelazo, P. D., Murphy, B., Durkin, F., Lister, M., & Masten, A. S. (2014). Promoting resilience through executive function training for homeless and highly mobile preschoolers. In S. Prince-Embury & D. H. Saklofske (Eds.), *Resilience interventions for youth in diverse populations* (pp. 133–158). Springer. https://doi.org/10.1007/978-1-4939-0542-3_7

Center on the Developing Child at Harvard University. (2011). *Construção do sistema de "Controle de Tráfego Aéreo" do cérebro: como as primeiras experiências moldam o desenvolvimento das funções executivas*. Relatório n. 11.

Dawson, P., & Guare, R. (2014). Interventions to promote executive development in children and adolescents. In S. Goldstein & J. A. Naglieri (Eds.), *Handbook of executive functioning* (pp. 427–444). Springer.

Diamond, A. (2013). Executive functions. *Annual Review of Psychology, 64*, 135–168. https://doi.org/10.1146/annurev-psych-113011-143750

Diamond, A., & Lee, K. (2011). Interventions shown to aid executive function development in children 4 to 12 years old. *Science, 333*(6045), 959–964. https://doi.org/10.1126/science.1204529

Diamond, A., Barnett, W. S., Thomas, J., & Munro, S. (2007). Preschool program improves cognitive control. *Science, 318*(5855), 1387–1388. https://doi.org/10.1126/science.1151148

Dias, N. M., & Seabra, A. G. (2013). *Programa de Intervenção em Autorregulação e Funções Executivas—PIAFEx*. Memnon.

Dias, N. M., & Seabra, A. G. (2015a). Is it possible to promote executive functions in preschoolers? A case study in Brazil. *International Journal of Child Care and Education Policy, 9*(6). https://doi.org/10.1186/s40723-015-0010-2

Dias, N. M., & Seabra, A. G. (2015b). The promotion of executive functioning in a Brazilian public school: A pilot study. *The Spanish Journal of Psychology, 18*, 1–14. https://doi.org/10.1017/sjp.2015.4

Dias, N. M., & Seabra, A. G. (2017). Intervention for executive functions development in early elementary school children: Effects on learning and behaviour, and follow-up maintenance. *Educational Psychology, 37*(4), 468–486. https://doi.org/10.1080/01443410.2016.1214686

Engel de Abreu, P. M. J., Abreu, N., Nikaedo, C. C., Puglisi, M. L., Tourinho, C. J., Miranda, M. C., Befi-Lopes, D. M., Bueno, O. F. A., & Martin, R. (2014a). Executive functioning and reading achievement in school: A study of Brazilian children assessed by their teachers as "poor readers". *Frontiers in Psychology, 5*, 550. https://doi.org/10.3389/fpsyg.2014.00550

Engel de Abreu, P. M. J., Nikaedo, C., Abreu, N., Tourinho, C. J., Miranda, M. C., Bueno, O. F. A., & Martin, R. (2014b). Working memory screening, school context, and socioeconomic status: An analysis of the effectiveness of the working memory rating scale in Brazil. *Journal of Attention Disorders, 18*(4), 346–356. https://doi.org/10.1177/1087054713476138

Evans, G. W., & Fuller-Rowell, T. E. (2013). Childhood poverty, chronic stress, and young adult working memory: The protective role of self-regulatory capacity. *Developmental Science, 16*(5), 688–696. https://doi.org/10.1111/desc.12082

Farah, M. J., Shera, D. M., Savage, J. H., Betancourt, L., Giannetta, J. M., Brodsky, N. L., Malmud, E. K., & Hurt, H. (2006). Childhood poverty: Specific associations with neurocognitive development. Brain Research, 1110(1), 166–174. https://doi.org/10.1016/j.brainres.2006.06.072.

Flook, L., Smalley, S. L., Kitil, M. J., Galla, B. M., Kaiser-Greenland, S., Locke, J., Ishijima, E., & Kasari, C. (2010). Effects of mindful awareness practices on executive functions in elementary school children. *Journal of Applied School Psychology, 26*(1), 70–95. https://doi.org/10.1080/15377900903379125

Freire, R. C. L. (2018). *PIAFEX-SD: Programa de Intervenção em Autorregulação e Funções Executivas para a Síndrome de Down* (Tese de Doutorado). Universidade Federal do Rio Grande do Norte.

Goldin, A. P., Hermida, M. J., Shalom, D. E., Elias Costa, M., Lopez-Rosenfeld, M., Segretin, M. S., Fernández-Slezak, D., Lipina, S. J., & Sigman, M. (2014). Far transfer to language and math of a short software-based gaming intervention. *Proceedings of the National Academy of Sciences of the United States of America, 111*(17), 6443–6448. https://doi.org/10.1073/pnas.1320217111

Guimarães, P., Tourinho, A., Vieira, J., & Alves, L. (2016). Uma Análise das possíveis contribuições do Gamebook Guardiões da Floresta para estimulação das funções executivas. XV Simpósio Brasileiro de Jogos e Entretenimento Digital. *Proceedings of SBGames, 2016*, 1165–1168.

Hackman, D. A., Gallop, R., Evans, G. W., & Farah, M. J. (2015). Socioeconomic status and executive function: Developmental trajectories and mediation. *Developmental Science, 18*(5), 686–702. https://doi.org/10.1111/desc.12246

Hornung, C., Schiltz, C., Brunner, M., & Martin, R. (2014). Predicting first-grade mathematics achievement: The contributions of domain-general cognitive abilities, nonverbal number sense, and early number competence. *Frontiers in Psychology, 5*, 1–18. https://doi.org/10.3389/fpsyg.2014.00272

Hughes, C. (2011). Changes and challenges in 20 years of research into the development of executive functions. *Infant & Child Development, 20*, 251–271.

Lima, R. F. (2015). *Programa de reabilitação neuropsicológica em funções executivas para estudantes com dislexia do desenvolvimento: elaboração e eficácia (Tese de Doutorado)*. Programa de pós-graduação em Ciências Médicas, Universidade Estadual de Campinas, Campinas, Brasil.

Lipina, S. J., Segretin, S., Hermida, J., Prats, L., Fracchia, C., Camelo, J. L., & Colombo, J. (2013). Linking childhood poverty and cognition: Environmental mediators of non-verbal executive control in an Argentine sample. *Developmental Science, 16*(5), 697–707. https://doi.org/10.1111/desc.12080

Meltzer, L. (2010). *Promoting executive functions in the classroom*. The Guilford Press.

Meltzer, L. (2014). Teaching executive functioning processes: Promoting metacognition, strategy use, and effort. In S. Goldstein & J. A. Naglieri (Eds.), *Handbook of executive functioning* (pp. 445–475). Springer.

Menezes, A., Dias, N. M., Trevisan, B. T., Carreiro, L. R. R., & Seabra, A. G. (2015). Intervention for executive functions in attention deficit and hyperactivity disorder. *Arquivos de Neuro-Psiquiatria, 73*(3), 227–236. https://doi.org/10.1590/0004-282X20140225

Miyake, A., Friedman, N. P., Emerson, M. J., Witzki, A. H., Howerter, A., & Wager, T. D. (2000). The unity and diversity of executive functions and their contributions to complex "Frontal Lobe" tasks: A latent variable analysis. *Cognitive Psychology, 41*(1), 49–100. https://doi.org/10.1006/cogp.1999.0734

Mulder, H., Verhagen, J., Van der Ven, S. H. G., Slot, P. L., & Leseman, P. P. M. (2017). Early executive function at age two predicts emergent mathematics and literacy at age five. *Frontiers in Psychology, 8*, 1–14. https://doi.org/10.3389/fpsyg.2017.01706

Nunes, L. G. (2017). *Abordagem Goal Management Training no desenvolvimento das funções executivas em adolescentes com queixas de disfunções executivas* (Dissertação de Mestrado). Universidade Presbiteriana Mackenzie.

Peijnenborgh, J. C. A. W., Hurks, P. M., Aldenkamp, A. P., Vles, J. S. H., & Hendriksen, J. G. M. (2016). Efficacy of working memory training in children and adolescents with learning disabilities: A review study and meta-analysis. *Neuropsychological Rehabilitation, 26*(5–6), 645–672. https://doi.org/10.1080/09602011.2015.1026356

Phillips, N. L., Mandalis, A., Benson, S., Parry, L., Epps, A., Morrow, A., & Lah, S. (2016). Computerized working memory training for children with moderate to severe traumatic brain injury: A double-blind, randomized, placebo-controlled trial. *Journal of Neurotrauma, 33*(23), 2097–2104. https://doi.org/10.1089/neu.2015.4358

Prince, M., Patel, V., Saxena, S., Mmaj, M., Maselko, J., Phillips, M., & Rahman, A. (2007). No health without mental health. *Lancet, 370*, 859–877.

Pureza, J. R., & Fonseca, R. P. (2016). *Cena – Programa de Capacitação de Educadores sobre Neuropsicologia da Aprendizagem com Ênfase em Funções Executivas e Atenção*. Ribeirão Preto: Booktoy.

Ramos, D. K. (2015). O uso da Escola do Cérebro no Ensino Fundamental: contribuições ao aprimoramento das habilidades cognitivas. *Anais do Seminário Tecnologias aplicadas a Educação e Saúde, 1*(1).

Ribner, A. D., Willoughby, M. T., & Blair, C. B. (2017). Executive function buffers the association between early math and later academic skills. *Frontiers in Psychology, 8*, 1–12. https://doi.org/10.3389/fpsyg.2017.00869

Riccio, C. A., & Gomes, H. (2013). Interventions for executive function deficits in children and adolescents. *Applied Neuropsychology: Child, 2*(2), 133–140.

Rocha, P., Filho, J. N., & Alves, L. (2014). Jogos digitais e reabilitação neuropsicológica: delineando novas mídias. *Anais do Seminário Tecnologias aplicadas a Educação e Saúde, 1*(1).

Roebers, C. M., Röthlisberger, M., Cimeli, P., Michel, E., & Neuenschwander, R. (2011). School enrolment and executive functioning: A longitudinal perspective on developmental changes, the influence of learning context, and the prediction of pre-academic skills. *European Journal of Developmental Psychology, 8*, 526–540.

Röthlisberger, M., Neuenschwander, R., Cimeli, P., Michel, E., & Roebers, C. M. (2012). Improving executive functions in 5- and 6-year-olds: Evaluation of a small group intervention in prekindergarten and kindergarten children. *Infant and Child Development, 21*(4), 411–429.

Sala, G., Aksayli, N. D., Tatlidil, K. S., Tatsumi, T., Gondo, Y., & Gobet, F. (2018). Near and far transfer in cognitive training: A second-order meta-analysis. *PsyArXiv, 26*.

Shayer, B., Carvalho, C. F., Mota, M., Argollo, N., Abreu, N., & Francisco, O. (2015). Desempenho de escolares em atenção e funções executivas no Nepsy e inteligência. *Psicologia: Teoria e Prática, 17*(1), 120–135. https://doi.org/10.15348/1980-6906/psicologia

Sohlberg, M. M., & Mateer, C. A. (2001). *Cognitive rehabilitation: An integrative neuropsychological approach*. Guilford Press.

Stelzer, F., Cervigni, M. A., & Martino, P. (2010). Bases neurales del desarrollo de las funciones ejecutivas durante la infancia y adolescencia. Una revisión. *Revista Chilena de Neuropsicología, 5*(54), 176–184.

Torres, V., & Alves, L. (2013). Professores e os jogos digitais: um olhar sobre as possibilidades pedagógicas destas mídias. *A Cor Das Letras, 14*(1), 163. https://doi.org/10.13102/cl.v14i1.1456

Van der Ven, S. H. G., Kroesbergen, E. H., Boom, J., & Leseman, P. P. M. (2012). The development of executive functions and early mathematics: A dynamic relationship. *British Journal of Educational Psychology, 82*(1), 100–119. https://doi.org/10.1111/j.2044-8279.2011.02035.x

Wu, K. K., Chan, S. K., Leung, P. W. L., Liu, W. S., Leung, F. L. T., & Ng, R. (2011). Components and developmental differences of executive functioning for school-aged children. *Developmental Neuropsychology, 36*(3), 319–337. https://doi.org/10.1080/87565641.2010.549979

Zito, J. M., Safer, D. J., dos Reis, S., Gardner, J. F., Boles, M., & Lynch, F. (2000). Trends in the prescribing of psychotropic medications to preschoolers. *JAMA, 283*, 1025–1030. https://doi.org/10.1001/jama.283.8.1025

Chapter 10
Considerations on Intervention in Theory of Mind in Childhood

Tatiana Pontrelli Mecca

Social cognition refers to processing social information or stimuli relevant to understanding individuals of the same species and their interactions (Happé et al., 2017). There has been an increase in studies over the years, especially in Social Neuroscience, which evidence the neurobiological substrates related to perception, manipulation, and response to social stimuli. Such findings relate various brain areas (ex, fusiform gyrus, amygdala, insula, superior temporal sulcus, superior temporal gyrus, prefrontal regions, among others) and neurotransmitters (ex, dopamine, serotonin, vasopressin, oxytocin, among others) to automatic and controlled processes that participate in social information processing (Cacioppo, 2016; Campanhã, 2016; Cozolino, 2014; Decety & Yoder; 2017; Happé & Frith, 2014; Mecca et al., 2016a; Rêgo et al., 2016; Spunt & Adolphs, 2017).

Unlike other constructs in psychology, few studies seek to understand the structure of Social Cognition, that is, what its components would be (Happé et al., 2017). This has a significant impact on intervention, as it should be directed at specific skills that allow social information processing. If, on the one hand, there is an accumulation of evidence about structural and functional aspects of the social brain, the definition of the components of social cognition lacks, therefore, investigation. Despite being scarce, there is some consensus among studies that the attribution of mental states, also called Theory of Mind, is among the skills that allow the individual to gain knowledge about the social world, recognizing it, interpreting it, and issuing appropriate responses to the context (Carruthers 2009; Fiske & Taylor, 2013; Green et al., 2015; Happé et al., 2017; Lewis & Todd 2005; Pinkham et al., 2014).

The attribution of mental states or Theory of Mind (ToM—from English *Theory of Mind*) refers to the ability to represent one's own and others' mental states

T. P. Mecca (✉)
Faculdade de Ciências Médicas da Santa Casa de São Paulo, São Paulo, Brazil
e-mail: tatiana.mecca@fcmsantacasasp.edu.br

C. O. Cardoso, N. M. Dias (eds.), *Neuropsychological Interventions for Children - Volume 1*, https://doi.org/10.1007/978-3-031-53586-4_10

(Happé et al., 2017). It is a system of inferences that allows understanding thoughts, emotions, desires, beliefs, memories, and intentions. This includes differentiating these implicit mental states among individuals and recognizing that they are not always compatible with reality but that they will guide one's own behavior and that of others (Mecca et al., 2018; Mecca et al., 2016b; Souza & Velludo, 2016).

This chapter will address the development and interventions in ToM, considering its preventive or promotional character in children with typical development as well as its remedial aspect in children with Autism Spectrum Disorder, one of the conditions in childhood that presents with ToM deficits.

Specific Domains of ToM

The importance of understanding the development and the need for interventions in ToM is due to the impact of this skill on adaptive functioning and mental health in childhood (Mecca et al., 2016; Ribeiro et al., 2016). There is evidence that the development of ToM is associated and predicts social competence, such as making friends and popularity among peers. It also relates to the involvement, use, and understanding of lying and deception, which are skills to play in a symbolic and imaginative way (Astington & Edward, 2010; Wellman, 2018).

Symbolic play is the game of make-believe; that is, it is the use of an object to represent another. For example, pretending to be a character or, during a game, being able to use an object, giving it a different function from the original, like using a spoon pretending to be a microphone or a phone (Astington & Edward, 2010; Bosa & Salles, 2018; Wellman, 2018). From the symbolic play, the child develops more complex skills, creating sequences structured in an associative and spontaneous way (Bosa & Salles, 2018). In this way, they are able to create characters and roles with stories that have a beginning, middle and end.

In addition to providing strategies for discussion, argumentation and persuasion in interaction with others (Wellman, 2018), ToM is related to lower rates of internalizing and externalizing behavior problems reported by parents and teachers (Gonçalves, 2017; Mecca et al., 2016). Nevertheless, relationships with academic performance and acceptance of *feedback* provided by teachers are also described (Wellman, 2018).

Various models regarding ToM are described in the literature as a broader domain, composed of specific skills/domains. This understanding is necessary since interventions can be directed at each aspect. Table 10.1 illustrates one of the first models, described by Premack (1988), in which the author divides ToM according to the characteristics of the stimuli.

According to this model, interventions could focus on the recognition and perception of emotions (Perceptive ToM), in promoting imitation or in sequencing actions according to the behavior of the other (Motivational ToM), in understanding the action of the other based on their desires, thoughts or beliefs (Informational ToM). Shamay-Tsoory et al. (2006) divide ToM into modules according to the type of attribution (Table 10.2).

Table 10.1 Premack's cognitive model (1988) for ToM

Perceptive ToM
Face processing Recognize other people's intentions based on their facial expressions
Motivational ToM
Observation of the other's actions Predisposition to follow the course of an action initiated by another
Informational ToM
Understanding the beliefs, desires, and thoughts of others Answers based on this understanding

Table 10.2 Modular perspective of ToM described by Shamay-Tsoory et al. (2006)

Affective ToM
Make attributions about feelings and emotions
Cognitive ToM
Make inferences about beliefs and causes of behaviors

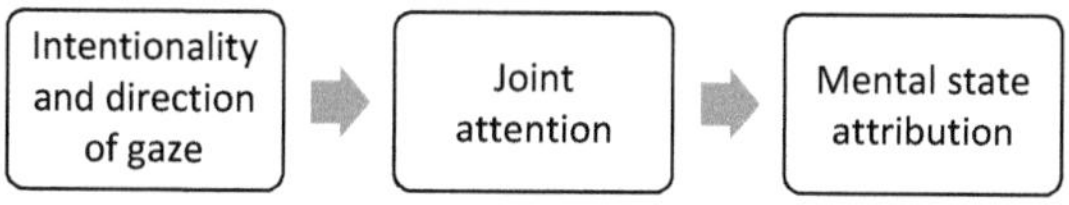

Fig. 10.1 Development modules of ToM according to Baron-Cohen (1995)

In the case of the description made by Shamay-Tsoory et al. (2006), the intervention could be directed at cognitive and affective aspects of ToM, considering the attributions made to one's own behavior and that of others. In addition to the models described, Baron-Cohen (1995) also studied individuals with ToM alterations, specifically Autism Spectrum Disorder (ASD), and made a functional division of ToM. For this, he considered its sequential development and precursor skills, as illustrated in Fig. 10.1.

The first module comprises two processes: intentionality, which refers to the recognition of the intention and desire that leads to an action, and the direction of gaze, which allows the understanding that when looking in the same direction as the other, both see the same stimulus. The integration of these two skills would lead to the joint attention, according to the second module (Baron-Cohen, 1995). Shared Attention is the ability to coordinate one's gaze with that of a social partner, which leads to sharing interests (Mundy et al., 2009).

Considered a precursor skill of ToM, shared attention has been one of the main targets of early intervention in children with sociocommunicative deficits, especially ASD. Early interventions in shared attention (Kasari et al., 2006; Zwaigenbaum et al., 2015) aim to develop both the initiative, which refers to the child's intention to share something with their social partner, and the response, characterized by understanding the communicative intentionality of the social partner (Bosa et al., 2016; Murza et al., 2016).

A meta-analysis conducted by Murza et al. (2016) assessed the efficacy of interventions in shared attention for children with ASD between 21 and 50 months. They evaluated 15 studies, in which interventions were conducted by parents, teachers, or undergraduate students, with duration ranging from 5 weeks to more than 6 months. The results showed improvements in the shared attention of children with ASD after the interventions. The effects occur regardless of who applies the intervention (parents, teachers, or professionals), the way the stimulation is carried out, the amount of stimulation received (in number of hours), or the type of study design, whether it is case-control or comparison between interventions that focus on shared attention or those that use symbolic play.

Part of the interventions carried out in ToM for individuals with ASD of different age groups focus on precursor skills (Fletcher-Watson et al., 2014; Murza et al., 2016). A review by Fletcher-Watson et al. (2014) showed that part of the interventions in ToM in ASD are directed at shared attention, imitation, and recognition of emotions.

Still on the different components of ToM, Tager-Flusberg and Sullivan (2000) describe it as a skill composed of two subsystems: socioperceptive and reflective. Both would be similar to what Premack (1988) called perceptual and motivational ToM (socioperceptive), and informational ToM (reflective system), as illustrated in Fig. 10.2.

In summary, the models present more similarities and convergences than opposing conceptions about ToM. They all conceive it as a broad domain composed of specific domains, these being the perception, recognition, and attribution of emotions; the recognition of intentionality and the purposeful action of the other; and the attribution of beliefs, desires, and thoughts, with reasoning and reflection on how these cause behaviors.

More recently, some authors have begun to study ToM, considering its implicit and explicit aspects. Implicit ToM refers to the ability to correctly anticipate an action based on an inference of the mental state of an agent, but without deliberately reflecting on this mental state. The literature reports this process as fast, automatic, and unconscious. Explicit ToM, on the other hand, is the conscious process of attributing mental states; it is flexible and deliberate, and the individual is able to reflect on it (Apperly & Butterfill, 2009; Frith & Frith, 2012).

Studies have indicated that individuals with ASD present more prominent deficits in implicit ToM, with impairments in looking ahead to stimuli that would

Subsystems	
Socioperceptive: Attributions of mental states based on facial expression, tone of voice and body movements	Reflective or socio-cognitive: Reasoning about mental states and behavior of others; integrates events over time

Fig. 10.2 Subsystems of ToM according to Tager-Flusberg and Sullivan (2000)

indicate the correct response in tasks of attributing mental states (Schuwerk et al., 2015; Senju, 2012). These results have relevant implications for intervention, since much of the knowledge about the effect of the Interventions in ToM for individuals with ASD is anchored in strategies for the development of explicit ToM.

Development of ToM

The development of ToM occurs in early stages (Wellman, 2014), with the stage from birth to 6 years being a sensitive period for the stimulation and promotion of this skill. Table 10.3 presents some general milestones of ToM development from childhood to adolescence according to a literature review by Souza and Velludo (2016), Astington and Edward (2010) and Wellman et al. (2001). This summary on the development of ToM can assist and guide the planning of interventions considering the normative characteristics expected for each stage.

Wellman et al. (2001) show that, in relation to the development of false belief, there is rapid growth during the preschool years and a decrease in growth rates after the age of 6. From this age, the increase in understanding of mental states is slower.

Table 10.3 Development of ToM from childhood to adolescence

Period	Developed skill
Newborns	Eye direction towards the mother's eyes; preference for social stimuli (faces and human voices).
First 6 months	Imitation of manual and facial gestures; social smile; response to sound.
From 9 to 12 months	Shared attention; cooperative interaction between baby, object and social partner; regulation of responses based on the caregiver's emotional reactions.
18 months	Manifests, verbally and non-verbally, own states of desires and emotions; attribution of intention in the action of others.
2 years	Understand that desires drive actions and that mental states are not observable or tangible. They make a connection between desire and emotion (ex, happy when they get something they want). Develop socioperceptive skills. Awareness that what they are thinking is different from what they see in the world (ex, symbolic play).
3 years	Children identify basic emotional expressions and understand that two individuals can have different desires and express emotions different from theirs in similar situations. Beginning of the reflective system and understanding of false belief.
4 years	Differentiate beliefs from desires. Understanding of false belief in development.
5 years	Understanding of false belief well established
From 6 years onwards	Demonstrate understanding that individuals can have internal emotions different from those expressed on their faces. Attribution of second-order beliefs onwards; understanding of irony and gaffes.
During adolescence	Use of complex attributions considering different contexts: their own mind and that of specific people with whom they interact, of strangers and of groups.

There are some differences between cultures during the evolution of false beliefs in relation to the beginning and period of development. However, there is evidence that in countries like the United States, United Kingdom, Canada, Australia, Austria, Japan, and Korea, the preschool years are periods of rapid growth and therefore more sensitive to interventions.

It is known that the development of ToM is related to a series of variables, among them the characteristics of the family environment and interaction with the caregiver and other family members, syntactic and semantic language, executive functions, time of schooling and interaction with peers (Astington & Jenkins, 1999; Batista et al., 2016; Mecca et al., 2016; Mello, 2018; Souza & Velludo, 2016; Wellman, 2018). Therefore, stimulating them can indirectly influence the promotion of ToM.

Investment in strategies and programs focused on ToM is necessary since deficits in this skill are associated with greater functional impairments (of adaptive behavior) in individuals with ASD. In typical children, there is evidence that worse scores on ToM tests at 5 years are related to higher rates of peer rejection at 6 and 7 years of age (Caputi et al., 2012), as well as reports of behavior problems by parents and teachers (Gonçalves, 2017).

Wellman (2018) synthesized the impact of ToM in the school environment. According to the author, this skill is associated with success in social circumstances that occur in school, such as peer acceptance, leadership, and grouping with other peers. It also relates to the use of metacognitive strategies and academic performance in reading, writing, and math. Finally, there is also a relationship with motivation for learning from persistence, the ability to deal with failures, and receive feedback from teachers. Given the impacts of impairments in ToM, the following section will discuss considerations about intervention

Interventions in Theory of Mind

Literature reviews in the area point out that interventions in ToM tend to be effective for those who receive them. This premise is true for both typical children and those with neurodevelopmental disorders, such as in the case of ASD (Zauza et al., 2016). Shorter training programs, in terms of the number of sessions, and longer sessions appear to have a greater effect (Hofmann et al., 2016). This information is promising in the sense that positive results can be observed in a short period of time.

Among the most used strategies, with proven efficacy, are conversation, storytelling, or even videos that allow highlighting and reflecting on the mental states of the characters. In this sense, shared and interactive reading promotes the understanding of social situations, actions of the characters, and discussion about the causes of their behaviors from thoughts, beliefs, desires, intentions, emotions, etc. (Ornaghi et al., 2014). Considering the use of conversation and narratives about mental states in interventions, it is necessary to highlight the important role of language. Parallel to specific ToM programs, it is recommended to stimulate semantic, syntactic, and pragmatic aspects of language.

Some activities about conversation and the use of stories can be found in the Intervention Program in Self-Regulation and Executive Functions—PIAFEx, for children at the end of Preschool and the beginning of Elementary School I. The program, whose objective is early and preventive intervention, is composed of 10 modules and one of them, module 5 includes conversation and storytelling activities whose objective is communication and conflict management (Dias & Seabra, 2013). The study showed that parents report, in the post-test and follow-up, fewer peer relationship problems and more pro-social behaviors in children who participated in the intervention with PIAFEx compared to children who did not receive the intervention (Dias & Seabra, 2017).

More recently, the Intervention Program for Self-Regulation Promotion—PIPA (Dias et al., 2015; León et al., 2023) was developed. Like PIAFEx, PIPA is intended for the last year of Preschool Education, whose intervention aims at prevention and development in preschool children. The program, applied by the teacher in the classroom, stimulates self-regulation with an emphasis on emotional regulation. Among the proposed activities are those for recognizing emotions, understanding emotions in contexts, and a specific module to develop emotional control and regulation skills. Efficacy studies of PIPA are still ongoing, but the partial data analyzed so far showed effects of the program on the development of ToM (Theory of Mind) (Almeida et al., 2018), improvement in measures of Regulation and Emotional Symptoms in children, according to scales filled out by teachers. In addition, an improvement in measures of stress and behavior promoting self-regulation in the classroom was identified in teachers (Zauza, 2018).

Although PIPA is not yet available, it was observed that activities based on processing and regulating emotions also favor ToM. Children who went through the program significantly improved in relation to controls regarding the ability to attribute basic emotions and the attribution of thoughts and beliefs (Almeida et al., 2018). One of the interesting findings of this study is that the control group had better emotion attribution skills compared to the experimental group before the intervention. After the intervention, the experimental group not only improved their ability to attribute emotions but their performance was significantly better than that of the control group.

As an example, one of the PIPA activities aims to promote the recognition of one's own emotions through children's drawings. A sheet is given with a drawing of the outline of a face, and the children must fill it with features of facial expression related to the emotion they are feeling at the moment. After the drawing, the teacher asks the children to form pairs and show their partner the emotion that was drawn, talk about it, and explain its characteristics and why they feel this way. Another activity aims at the development of emotional regulation. Vignettes (short stories) are presented and then the teacher asks some questions about the actions and feelings of the characters so that the children understand the consequences of behaviors and the importance of thinking before acting or speaking.

Specifically in cases of ASD, a review showed the use of different strategies, such as the use of computerized programs or cartoons for emotion recognition training, one-to-one method (e.g., therapist-patient or teacher-student) in non-computerized activities, using figures and images so that from the context, the child can infer their mental states (beliefs, desires, and emotions). Some studies also used this strategy but with interventions for groups. Others were conducted based on parent-child activities and interaction. Generally, most lasted from two weeks to six months, and time varied from 30 minutes to 3 hours and 50 minutes per week (Fletcher-Watson et al., 2014).

Among the specific activities to develop ToM, the literature refers to the use of the testing paradigms themselves, that is, situations or vignettes in which the child must infer the character's mental state. Some of the testing paradigms also used in the intervention are described in Table 10.4. The reader can access the tasks described in Oliveira and Mecca (2016), Mecca (2018), Mecca et al. (2018), Mecca and Dias (2017), and Wellman and Liu (2004).

Fletcher-Watson et al. (2014) observed a significant increase in the target skill of interventions (for example, imitation, imaginative play, emotion recognition, shared attention, and false belief attribution). However, it seems that there is little evidence of generalization of gains to different contexts or maintenance of them over a long period of time. Another aspect discussed is that the level of evidence of the efficacy of ToM interventions in ASD is low; that is, there are limitations of sample selection, lack of blind evaluation of the effects of the intervention, participants are also not blind to the objectives of the interventions carried out and of the pre and post-intervention evaluations, as well as limitations of outcome measures and ways of reporting results.

In general, the promotion of orientation to social stimuli (smile, voice, gaze), shared attention, imitation, symbolic play, naming and recognition of emotions, use

Table 10.4 Theory of Mind tasks in the ascending order of difficulty

Task	Task objective
Diverse Desire	Verify if the child understands that the character has a desire different from their own.
Diverse Belief	Verify if the child understands that the character has a belief different from their own. In this case, there is not yet a true or false belief.
Access to Knowledge	Verify if the child understands that the character has knowledge different from their own.
False Content Belief	Verify if the child understands that the character has a belief that does not correspond with reality.
Explicit False Belief	Verify if the child infers the behavior of the character, knowing that they have a belief different from reality.
Emotion and Belief	Verify if the child understands the character's emotion upon experiencing disappointment.
Real Emotion × Apparent Emotion	Verify if the child understands that a character can feel and display one emotion.

Source: Adapted from Wellman and Liu (2004)

of narratives and storytelling with active participation of children, as well as tasks based on testing paradigms can contribute to the development of ToM, although it is still unknown how long the effect of the intervention remains and whether the knowledge acquired is generalized to different contexts in children with atypical development. On the other hand, the results are more favorable with typical children and future studies are needed to fill this gap in relation to the effects of ToM interventions in ASD.

References

Almeida, A. A., Maioli, M. C. P., León, C. R. B., Seabra, A. G., Dias, N. M., & Mecca. T. P. (2018). Promoção da Autorregulação em pré-escolares: efeito sobre a Teoria da Mente. Pôster apresentado no Congress on Brain, Behaviors and Emotions 2018. Gramado, RS.

Apperly, I. A., & Butterfill, S. A. (2009). Do humans have two systems to track beliefs and belief-like states? *Psychological Review, 116*(4), 953. https://doi.org/10.1037/a0016923

Astington, J. W., & Edward, M. J. (2010). The development of theory of mind in early childhood. *Social Cognition in Infancy, 5*, 16.

Astington, J. W., & Jenkins, J. M. (1999). A longitudinal study of the relation between language and theory-of-mind development. *Developmental Psychology, 35*(5), 1311. https://doi.org/10.1037/0012-1649.35.5.1311

Baron-Cohen, S. (1995). *Mindblindness. Na essay in autism and theory of mind.* The MIT Press.

Batista, L. S., Martins, G. L. L., Seabra, A. G., & Dias, N. M. (2016). Teoria da mente: relações e predição a partir das funções executivas. In T. P. Mecca, N. M. Dias, & A. A. Berberian (Eds.), *Cognição Social: Teoria pesquisa e aplicação* (pp. 78–89). Memnon.

Bosa, C. A., & Salles, J. F. (2018). *Protea-R: Sistema de Avaliação da Suspeita de Transtorno do Espectro Autista.* Vetor Editora.

Bosa, C. A., Zanon, R. B., & Backes, B. (2016). Autismo: construção do protocolo de avaliação do comportamento da criança-PROTEA-R. *Revista Psicologia Teoria e Prática, 18*(1), 194–205. https://doi.org/10.15348/1980-6906

Cacioppo, J. T. (2016). *Social neuroscience.* MIT Press.

Campanhã, C. (2016). O papel da cognição social na tomada de decisão. In T. P. Mecca, N. M. Dias, & A. A. Berberian (Eds.), *Cognição Social: Teoria, Pesquisa e Aplicação* (pp. 100–109). Editora Memnon.

Caputi, M., Lecce, S., Pagnin, A., & Banerjee, R. (2012). Longitudinal effects of theory of mind on later peer relations: The role of prosocial behavior. *Developmental Psychology, 48*(1), 257. https://doi.org/10.1037/a0025402

Carruthers, P. (2009). How we know our own minds: the relationship between mindreading and metacognition. *Behavioral and Brain Sciences, 32*(2), 121–138. https://doi.org/10.1017/S0140525X09000545

Cozolino, L. (2014). *The neuroscience of human relationships: Attachment and the developing social brain.* WW Norton & Company.

Decety, J., & Yoder, K. J. (2017). The emerging social neuroscience of justice motivation. *Trends in Cognitive Sciences, 21*(1), 6–14. https://doi.org/10.1016/j.tics.2016.10.008

Dias, N. M., & Seabra, A. G. (2013). *Programa de Intervenção em Autorregulação e Funções Executivas – PIAFEx.* Memnon.

Dias, N. M., & Seabra, A. G. (2017). Intervention for executive functions development in early elementary school children: effects on learning and behaviour, and follow-up maintenance. *Educational Psychology, 37*(4), 468–486. https://doi.org/10.1080/01443410.2016.1214686

Dias, N. M., Mecca, T. P., León, C. R., Zauza, G., Muniz, M., & Seabra, A. G. (2015). Programa de Intervenção para Promoção de Autorregulação – PIPA.
Fiske, S. T., & Taylor, S. E. (2013). *Social cognition: From brains to culture*. Sage.
Fletcher-Watson, S., McConnell, F., Manola, E., & McConachie, H. (2014). Interventions based on the Theory of Mind cognitive model for autism spectrum disorder (ASD). *Cochrane Database of Systematic Reviews, 3*, CD008785. https://doi.org/10.1002/14651858.CD008785.pub2
Frith, C. D., & Frith, U. (2012). Mechanisms of social cognition. *Annual Review of Psychology, 63*, 287–313. https://doi.org/10.1146/annurev-psych-120710-100449
Gonçalves, B. (2017). Relação entre Teoria da Mente e índices comportamentais em crianças pré-escolares. (Dissertação de Mestrado). Centro Universitário Fieo, Osasco.
Green, M. F., Horan, W. P., & Lee, J. (2015). Social cognition in schizophrenia. *Nature Reviews Neuroscience, 16*(10), 620.
Happé, F., & Frith, U. (2014). Annual research review: Towards a developmental neuroscience of atypical social cognition. *Journal of Child Psychology and Psychiatry, 55*(6), 553–577. https://doi.org/10.1111/jcpp.12162
Happé, F., Cook, J. L., & Bird, G. (2017). The structure of social cognition: In(ter) dependence of sociocognitive processes. *Annual Review of Psychology, 68*, 243–267. https://doi.org/10.1146/annurev-psych-010416-044046
Hofmann, S. G., Doan, S. N., Sprung, M., Wilson, A., Ebesutani, C., Andrews, L. A., Curtiss, J., & Harris, P. L. (2016). Training children's theory-of-mind: A meta-analysis of controlled studies. *Cognition, 150*, 200–212. https://doi.org/10.1016/j.cognition.2016.01.006
Kasari, C., Freeman, S., & Paparella, T. (2006). Joint attention and symbolic play in young children with autism: A randomized controlled intervention study. *Journal of Child Psychology and Psychiatry, 47*(6), 611–620. https://doi.org/10.1111/j.1469-7610.2005.01567.x
Leon, C. B. R., Mecca, T. P., Muniz, M., Seabra, A. G., Zauza, G., & Dias, N. M. (2023). Desenvolvimento do Programa de Intervenção para Promoção de Autorregulação Infantil. *Psicopedagogia, 40*, 204–219.
Lewis, M. D., & Todd, R. M. (2005). Getting emotional: A neural perspective on emotion, intention, and consciousness. *Journal of Consciousness Studies, 12*(8-9), 210–235.
Mecca, T. P. (2018). Avaliação da Teoria da Mente no pré-escolar. In N. M. Dias & A. G. Seabra (Eds.), *Neuropsicologia com pré-escolares. Coleção Neuropsicologia na Prática Clínica* (pp. 135–148). Pearson.
Mecca, T. P., & Dias, N. M. (2017). Avaliação de Cognição Social no Transtorno do Espectro Autista. In C. A. Bosa & M. C. T. V. Teixeira (Eds.), *Autismo: avaliação psicológica e neuropsicológica* (pp. 119–134). Hogrefe.
Mecca, T. P., Dias, N. M., & Berberian, A. A. (2016a). Cognição Social. In Mecca, N. M. Dias, & A. A. Berberian (Eds.), *Cognição Social: Teoria, Pesquisa e Aplicação* (pp. 10–23). Editora Memnon.
Mecca, T. P., Gonçalves, B., Pontes, J. M., & Dias, N. M. (2016b). Cognição Social: Relação com variáveis ambientais e desfechos comportamentais. In T. P. Mecca, N. M. Dias, & A. A. Berberian (Eds.), *Cognição Social: Teoria, Pesquisa e Aplicação* (pp. 90–99). Editora Memnon.
Mecca, T. P., Dias, N. M., Oliveira, P. V., & Muniz, M. (2018). Teste de Teoria da Mente para Crianças: Validade de Conteúdo. *Psico-Usf, 23*(3), 393–407. https://doi.org/10.1590/1413-82712018230301
Mello, D. P. (2018). Relação entre Teoria da Mente e nível socioeconômico em crianças de 4 a 7 anos de idade. (Dissertação de Mestrado). Centro Universitário Fieo, Osasco.
Mundy, P., Sullivan, L., & Mastergeorge, A. M. (2009). A parallel and distributed-processing model of joint attention, social cognition and autism. *Autism Research, 2*(1), 2–21. https://doi.org/10.1002/aur.61
Murza, K. A., Schwartz, J. B., Hahs-Vaughn, D. L., & Nye, C. (2016). Joint attention interventions for children with autism spectrum disorder: a systematic review and meta-analysis. *International Journal of Language & Communication Disorders, 51*(3), 236–251. https://doi.org/10.1111/1460-6984.12212

Oliveira, P. V., & Mecca, T. P. (2016). Ferramentas para avaliação de teoria da mente na infância. In T. P. Mecca, N. M. Dias, & A. A. Berberian (Eds.), *Cognição Social: Teoria, Pesquisa e Aplicação* (pp. 110–125). Editora Memnon.

Ornaghi, V., Brockmeier, J., & Grazzani, I. (2014). Enhancing social cognition by training children in emotion understanding: A primary school study. *Journal of Experimental Child Psychology, 119*, 26–39. https://doi.org/10.1016/j.jecp.2013.10.005

Pinkham, A. E., Penn, D. L., Green, M. F., Buck, B., Healey, K., & Harvey, P. D. (2014). The social cognition psychometric evaluation study: results of the expert survey and RAND Panel. *Schizophrenia Bulletin, 40*(4), 813–823. https://doi.org/10.1093/schbul/sbt081

Premack, D. (1988). 'Does the chimpanzee have a theory of mind' revisited. In R. W. Byrne & A. Whiten (Eds.), *Machiavellian intelligence: social expertise and the evolution of intellect in monkeys, apes, and humans* (pp. 160–179). Oxford University Press.

Rêgo, G. G., Valasek, C. A., Marques, L. M., & Boggio, P. S. (2016). Contribuições das neurociências para a compreensão da cognição social. In T. P. Mecca, N. M. Dias, & A. A. Berberian (Eds.), *Cognição Social: Teoria, Pesquisa e Aplicação* (pp. 54–69). Memnon.

Ribeiro, S., Silva, M. C. S., Araripe, B., Gome, M. T., Bordini, D., & Cunha, G. R. (2016). Cognição Social e Saúde Mental. In T. P. Mecca, N. M. Dias, & A. A. Berberian (Eds.), *Cognição Social: Teoria, Pesquisa e Aplicação* (pp. 188–197). Memnon.

Schuwerk, T., Vuori, M., & Sodian, B. (2015). Implicit and explicit theory of mind reasoning in autism spectrum disorders: The impact of experience. *Autism, 19*(4), 459–468. https://doi.org/10.1177/1362361314526004

Senju, A. (2012). Spontaneous theory of mind and its absence in autism spectrum disorders. *The Neuroscientist, 18*(2), 108–113. https://doi.org/10.1177/1073858410397208

Shamay-Tsoory, S. G., Tibi-Elhanany, Y., & Aharon-Peretz, J. (2006). The ventromedial prefrontal cortex is involved in understanding affective but not cognitive theory of mind stories. *Social Neuroscience, 1*(3–4), 149–166. https://doi.org/10.1080/17470910600985589

Souza, D. H., & Velludo, N. (2016). O Desenvolvimento da Teoria da Mente. In T. P. Mecca, N. M. Dias, & A. A. Berberian (Eds.), *Cognição Social: Teoria, Pesquisa e Aplicação* (pp. 42–53). Editora Memnon.

Spunt, R. P., & Adolphs, R. (2017). A new look at domain specificity: insights from social neuroscience. *Nature Reviews Neuroscience, 18*(9), 559.

Tager-Flusberg, H., & Sullivan, K. (2000). A componential view of theory of mind: evidence from Williams syndrome. *Cognition, 76*(1), 59–90. https://doi.org/10.1016/S0010-0277(00)00069-X

Wellman, H. M. (2014). *Making minds: How theory of mind develops*. Oxford University Press.

Wellman, H. M. (2018). Theory of mind: The state of the art. European Journal of Developmental Psychology, 1–29. doi: https://doi.org/10.1080/17405629.2018.1435413

Wellman, H. M., & Liu, D. (2004). Scaling of theory-of-mind tasks. *Child Development, 75*(2), 523–541. https://doi.org/10.1111/j.1467-8624.2004.00691.x

Wellman, H. M., Cross, D., & Watson, J. (2001). Meta-analysis of theory-of-mind development: The truth about false belief. *Child development, 72*(3), 655–684. https://doi.org/10.1111/1467-8624.00304

Zauza, G. (2018). Programa de Intervenção para Promoção de Autorregulação: análise de efeitos em pré-escolares e seus professores. (Dissertação de Mestrado). Centro Universitário FIEO, Osasco.

Zauza, G., Mecca, T. P., & Dias, N. M. (2016). Promoção do desenvolvimento da Teoria da Mente: modelos de intervenção e evidências. In T. P. Mecca, N. M. Dias, & A. A. Berberian (Eds.), *Cognição Social: Teoria, Pesquisa e Aplicação* (pp. 138–151). editora Memnon.

Zwaigenbaum, L., Bauman, M. L., Choueiri, R., Kasari, C., Carter, A., Granpeesheh, D., Mailloux, Z., Roley, S. S., Wagner, S., Fein, D., Pierce, K., Buie, T., Davis, P. A., Newschaffer, C., Robins, D., Wetherby, A., Stone, W. L., Yirmiya, N., Estes, A., Hansen, R. L., McPartland, J. C., Natowicz, M. R., & Pierce, K. (2015). Early intervention for children with autism spectrum disorder under 3 years of age: recommendations for practice and research. *Pediatrics, 136*(Supplement 1), S60–S81.

Chapter 11
Stimulation and Neuropsychological Rehabilitation of Social and Emotional Skills in Childhood

Nara Côrtes Andrade and Chrissie Ferreira de Carvalho

Social and Emotional Skills in Childhood: Debating Constructs

In childhood, emotional, social, and cognitive development are intertwined more intensely than in other stages of development. The first tool of human communication, emotions color and give meaning to socialization and cognitive processes. They are central to peer relationships and well-being and are linked to understanding the world and the sense of *self*. From birth, babies share their internal states with their social partners and are capable of processing information related to the affective state of the same (Bergamasco, 1997). Skills such as imitation, perception, and communication are found in newborns (Ribeiro et al., 2004). According to Bussab and Ribeiro (1998), human beings are biologically cultural. Therefore, understanding the basis of social behavior and human emotional development is essential for individuals with typical development and neuropsychiatric disorders (Järvinen et al., 2013).

Elias and collaborators (1997, cited by Durlak et al., 2011) define Social and Emotional Learning (SEL) as the development of core competencies to recognize and manage emotions, establish and achieve positive goals, deal constructively with conflicts, understand and demonstrate empathetic behaviors with social partners, establish and maintain positive relationships, as well as make ethical and responsible decisions. The socioemotional ability refers, therefore, to the ability and motivation to act, think, and feel in socially responsible ways.

N. C. Andrade
Universidade Federal de Juiz de Fora, Juiz de Fora, Brazil
e-mail: nara.andrade@ufjf.br

C. F. de Carvalho (✉)
Universidade Federal de Santa Catarina, Florianópolis, Brazil
e-mail: chrissie.carvalho@ufsc.br

C. O. Cardoso, N. M. Dias (eds.), *Neuropsychological Interventions for Children - Volume 1*, https://doi.org/10.1007/978-3-031-53586-4_11

Emotions are complex and multidimensional and occur in response to significant life events (challenges or opportunities) in each individual's external or internal environment. They always influence what we perceive, think, and do, playing an important motivational and informative role (Izard, 2009). They form the basis of temperament and personality, considering the stability of patterns of emotional responses in the face of a constantly changing environment (Izard, 2002). Emotions widely influence cognitive and behavioral processes, constituting social and moral behavior. They play a significant role in empathy and the ability to understand mental states, among other aspects of social skills. Their brain processing is not restricted to subcortical regions, which are more primitive in terms of phylogenetic development. Emotions also "recruit portions of the frontal lobe, which is the largest and most recent brain structure to develop in the human brain" (Peretz, 2009, p. 100). In a meta-analysis conducted on the functional neuroanatomy of emotions, Phan et al. (2002) corroborated the role of the medial prefrontal cortex in the neurocircuitry of emotions. According to Liotti and Panksepp (2004, p. 35), "cortico-subcortical interactions create a special richness for human emotional life, as well as existential forms of emotional turbulences, unknown in other species."

Emotional comprehension (EC) encompasses multiple dimensions: the ability to recognize emotions in various contexts—signals in facial expressions, vocal, body language, and musical; labeling and naming emotions; identifying the causes or triggers of emotions in oneself and others; understanding the relationships between emotion, motivation, and behavior; recognizing dissimulation, co-occurrence, and ambivalence of emotions (Izard, 2001). EC promotes the development of a healthy relationship between the individual and their context as it assists in anticipating other people's feelings and behaviors and expressing one's own feelings.

Emotional regulation (ER) refers to intrinsic and extrinsic processes involved in evaluating, monitoring, and modifying psychophysiological reactions related to emotions in relation to personal goals (Arango, 2007). Regulating emotions allows them to be at an optimal excitatory level to facilitate their healthy use in a social context (Izard et al., 2008b). The set of processes in which emotions are regulated is heterogeneous and involves decreasing the intensity of an emotion, increasing the intensity of an emotion, or maintaining an ongoing emotion (Gross, 2007). The modifications can occur, for example, in terms of emotional dynamics, latency, duration, or magnitude. ER is closely related to numerous dimensions of social functioning, such as empathy, pro-social behavior, and aggression (Denham et al., 2012; Eisenberg et al., 2010). According to (Izard et al., 2008a, p. 371), ER "facilitates the use of cognitive and action systems to respond effectively to challenges and opportunities." It enables, for example, the child to think through conflict situations and to analyze the point of view of the other person with whom they are interacting. Children with difficulty in ER have little awareness about how and when to properly express their emotions (Eisenberg et al., 1994). Impairments in this skill have social implications and for the relationship between peers. Unable to communicate their emotions, divert their attention or think through their actions, children may respond to devastating feelings of stress by engaging in non-adaptive behaviors (Izard et al., 2008b). They may use externalizing strategies, such as hetero-aggression and hostile responses or internalizing strategies, such as excessive worry about an event, avoidance of social contact, or blaming oneself. Bryant (1998, cited by Izard, 2002, p. 204) states that "children often resort to ineffective coping mechanisms because they have little experience with more effective strategies."

Emotional comprehension (EC) and regulation (ER) are fundamental for managing and using emotions in a healthy way (Trentacosta & Fine, 2010). They are related to numerous and important dimensions of human cognitive and socio-affective functioning and having a close relationship with each other. Research indicates positive correlations between EC and ER with inhibitory control skills (Morgan et al., 2010), social skills (Miller et al., 2005; Schultz et al., 2001), conflict resolution (Liao et al., 2014), and academic skills (Bennett et al., 2005; Trentacosta & Izard, 2007). At the same time, impairments in EC and ER are related to higher levels of aggression (Denham et al., 2002), behavioral problems and negative peer interactions (Miller et al., 2005; Morgan et al., 2010).

Promotion of Social and Emotional Skills and Mental Health Prevention in Childhood

Social and Emotional Learning (SEL) programs combine methodologies seeking to integrate emotion, cognition, communication, and behavior (Lemerise & Arsenio, 2000). Among their main objectives is the development of competencies: self-awareness, self-regulation, relationship skills, social awareness, and responsible decision-making (Durlak et al., 2011). According to Izard, King, and collaborators (2008a), interventions for SEL aim to reduce risk and increase protective factors in development. SEL interventions occur in various contexts and can be grouped into: (1) programs developed before school entry, (2) programs developed in a school context, and (3) programs developed after school (Puerta et al., 2016). In this chapter, we will present interventions aimed at the school context.

The structuring of curricula and interventions in school environments at any age, including during Early Childhood Education, focuses on cognitive and linguistic dimensions, with few curricula explicitly addressing the social and emotional dimensions (Denham, 1998). However, socio-emotional skills establish the basis for the construction of social relationships among peers and teachers and promote positive relationships, helping to create a positive and favorable climate for the learning process in the classroom. Since the 1950s, programs have been developed to prevent social and behavioral problems (Durlak & Wells, 1997). In the 90s, programs seeking to improve mental health in the school environment expanded in the United States but are still little disseminated in other locations (Izard et al., 2002). A publication by the World Bank analyzed 86 SEL programs in various contexts and age groups from 17 countries, reporting only two programs in Brazil, for example, both outside the school context and with an emphasis on adolescents and young adults (Puerta et al., 2016).

There is an effort by the scientific community to evaluate the efficacy of programs for the promotion of SEL, reflected in various studies, such as the meta-analysis carried out by Durlak and collaborators (2011) evaluating 213 SEL programs and 250,000 children and adolescents in a school context or the publication made in 2016, by the World Bank (Puerta et al., 2016). The literature indicates that the stimulation of social and emotional skills contributes to improving skills of emotional comprehension (Domitrovich et al., 2007; Izard et al., 2008a); and emotional regulation and stress management (Domitrovich et al., 2007; Durlak et al., 2011; Izard et al., 2008a; Kraag et al., 2006; Sprung et al., 2015); social competence, problem-solving skills, empathy, and pro-social behavior (Domitrovich et al., 2007; Durlak et al., 2011; Frey et al., 2005; Izard et al., 2008a; Sprung et al., 2015); self-efficacy and decision-making skills (Durlak et al., 2011); increasing expressions of positive emotions and decreasing negative expressions evaluated by teachers (Izard et al., 2008a); reducing aggressive behaviors, externalizing and internalizing behavior problems (Durlak & Wells, 1997; Frey et al., 2005; Izard et al., 2008a), in addition to contributing to engagement in classroom activities, academic performance (Durlak et al., 2011; Durlak & Wells, 1997) and economic and labor outcomes in adult life (Puerta et al., 2016).

Emotions are the most relevant elements during childhood to motivate thoughts and actions (Izard et al., 2008a). Positive emotions increase sociability, well-being, and constructive behavior (Izard, 2002). They are a constant element in children's games and play. Playing, the ultimate expression of childhood, is essential to the development of social and emotional skills, as well as cognitive and motor skills. At the same time, joy benefits cognitive processes of memory and learning, increasing cognitive flexibility, curiosity, and the exploration of new coping alternatives to situations (Fernández-Abascal et al., 2010). Joy favors interpersonal relationships and bond establishment, increasing the ability to enjoy various aspects of life, enabling the generalization of positive attitudes and, consequently the emergence of empathetic and altruistic behaviors (Fernandéz-Abascal et al., 2010). In addition to expanding the repertoire of thoughts and actions that favor coping with negative life events and increase resilience (Fredrickson & Levenson, 1998), Joy is also an important element for consolidating self-esteem in situations of achievement in performing a task. ASE programs can timely introduce new and challenging stimuli and activities that, age-appropriate, could activate interest and motivation and also facilitate experiences of success that activate joy (Izard, 2002)

ASE stimulation programs can also emphasize the development of empathy and pro-social behavior. Teaching children to understand their own emotions and the emotions of others, as well as the point of view, allows for a greater number of empathetic responses and, consequently, pro-social behaviors (Izard, 2002). According to Izard (2002), recognizing emotional expressions of sadness, for example, favors the emergence of empathetic and altruistic behaviors towards those experiencing this emotion. At the same time, the empathetic response also activates the emotion of sadness and reduces aggressive reactions from peers. Therefore, It is essential to provide opportunities for the child to name emotions, compare different expressions of emotions in their various intensities, and provide activities that increase the skills to decode emotional signals and recognize expressions of emotion.

Understanding the causes and consequences of emotions favors the development of skills in other domains of social cognition. Games about the relationships between situations, causes, and consequences of emotions allow the child to perceive that each individual has a different emotionality and can respond differently to situations (Izard et al., 2008b). This understanding is important for developing the theory of mind and being one of the bases for empathy and pro-social behavior. It is also important to stimulate the child to generate dialogues and verbalizations about emotional situations, in addition to providing a welcoming atmosphere in the classroom that encourages a sense of belonging to the group and respect for the diversity of each child. Literature, as well as reference adults, can be important elements for the stimulation of pro-social behavior.

The ability to name emotions and "put feelings into words" is one of the first emotional schemes that emerge during childhood. Around 18 months, children begin to use language to meet their own emotional needs and to make associations between the emotions expressed by others and their desires (Bosacki & Moore, 2004). It is very important for the child to talk about their emotions and those of others (Bosacki & Moore, 2004). Emotional expressions enable the conceptualization of emotions, providing children with a rich tool to understand emotions. The possibility of expressing emotions and feelings verbally favors the reduction of crying in anger, as it provides children with a new way to express themselves, benefiting the development of understanding and emotional regulation (Coll et al., 2004; Morgan et al., 2010). Language has a critical regulatory function for emotions, as it allows for the verbal expression of feelings and the resolution of conflicts, in addition to the child using it in self-talk, promoting self-awareness, and self-regulation.

ASE programs dedicate a significant part of their methodologies to the regulation of negative emotions and stress management. Although the activation of negative emotions potentially increases the chance of maladaptive behaviors, when modulated, they also provide an opportunity to learn how to use the energy and motivation of this emotion constructively (Izard, 2002). Modulating the intensity or duration of emotional states, instead of suppressing intense emotions, with the constructive redirection of the motivational energy of the emotion is healthy. The suppression or denial of feelings also referred to as avoidance, contributes to triggering an increase in emotional arousal, intensifying the emotional experience. On the other hand, emotion modulation produces positive benefits, especially if coordinated with cognitive-emotional restructuring (Izard et al., 2008b). A series of emotional regulation strategies are used in dealing with negative emotions and stress (Izard, 2009; Izard et al., 2008b). Table 11.1 summarizes four emotional regulation strategies: active coping, social support, distraction, and avoidance.

The turtle technique, proposed by Robin, Schneider, and Dolnick in 1976 (cited by Domitrovich et al., 2007), is used in revised versions in various programs, such as the Intervention Program in Self-Regulation and Executive Functions—PIAFEx (Dias & Seabra, 2013). It encourages emotional modulation. This technique encourages children to return to their "turtle shell" when feeling hurt or angry. While they

Table 11.1 Strategies for regulation and coping with negative emotions and stress

Active coping
Ability to perceive the event as controllable, seeking to change the source of stress. Ability to perceive that the solution to the event is not feasible and to use cognitive strategies, such as: 1. Cognitive restructuring: a strategy that involves reassessing a situation in a more positive way, minimizing its unpleasant aspects or trying to find some meaning in it. 2. Constructive thinking: thinking of a way to solve everyday problems, for example, interpreting a situation as a challenge and not as a threat or perceiving a failure as a temporary setback instead of a definitive life sentence.
Social support
Asking others for help to directly handle a situation. By sharing their negative feelings, the child may feel more welcomed, and this action brings comfort. Younger children usually seek help from their parents, while the older ones seek support from their peers.
Distraction
It is characterized as an active effort to divert attention, that is, to take the problem off the mind and seek pleasurable activities such as playing, watching television, or listening to music. It is important to recognize negative feelings before seeking a substitute. Distraction has a regulatory function, as it reduces the initial arousal of stressful and negative feelings and calms the child. One can actively think of another positive emotion to change the focus that is causing discomfort, stress, or frustration.
Avoidance
It is characterized by the action of suppression or denial of unpleasant feelings without replacing them with a pleasant action.

Adapted from Izard (2004)

are in the "shell," they can reflect on their feelings and think about the best way to react to what or who caused these feelings. At this point, the child emerges from their "turtle shell." Other ER techniques are described in the literature. An example is the hold tight technique or hug technique (Izard, 2002). This technique, based on the Differential Theory of Emotions, seeks to facilitate the child's use of some of the arousal energy of anger to negotiate and resolve the eliciting situation, in addition to using language as a complementary strategy for emotional regulation and conflict resolution encouraging the expression of the feeling of emotion (Izard et al., 2008b). Both techniques modulate the arousal of anger and use breathing strategies to decrease the action of the autonomic nervous system. Table 11.2 summarizes the steps of the turtle technique and hug techniques' steps (Hold Tight).

In addition to the sessions of systematized intervention, it is important that teachers are trained to facilitate the understanding and regulation of emotions in children during their occurrence, whether in games and play or in other situations. This allows the child to learn to name their emotional states, regulate their emotions, and engage in discourse about their emotions and functions in a protected environment. ASE strategies are presented in Table 11.3 of this chapter.

Table 11.2 Examples of emotional regulation techniques

Turtle technique[a]		Hug technique[b]
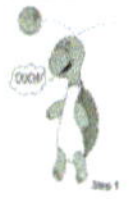	Step 1: Recognize your feeling(s)	Step 1: Hug yourself or something soft and take three deep breaths, counting the breaths
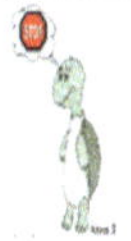	Step 2: Think about "stopping"	Step 2: Use your words. Say what the problem is
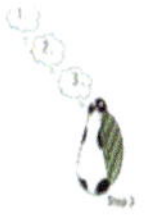	Step 3: Go inside your "shell" and take three deep breaths	Step 3: Wait and listen to the other child
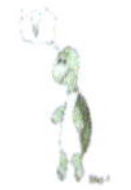	Step 4: Come out of the shell and, when you are calm, think of a "solution"	Step 4: Talk about the issue and find a way to play fair

[a]Adapted from Domitrovich et al. (2007)
[b]Adapted from Izard, Stark et al. (2008b)

Social Emotional Learning Programs in the School Context

There is evidence of a larger effect size in programs developed in early childhood (Durlak et al., 2011; Durlak & Wells, 1997; Puerta et al., 2016), suggesting that this is a period especially sensitive for preventive interventions for social and emotional and behavioral problems. Meta-analyses indicate that the quality of program implementation and the duration and intensity of the intervention have a significant moderating effect on the results of the same. Durlak et al. (2011) recommend that the practices developed adopt four pillars: adopt a sequential, step-by-step learning approach, use active methodologies based on activities, dedicate sufficient time to skill development, and make explicit learning objectives. These are the principles of the SAFE approach, that is, Sequenced, Active, Focused, and Explicit programs, pointed out in the literature as a strategy that favors the effectiveness of programs (Durlak et al., 2011; Puerta et al., 2016). Puerta et al. (2016) also emphasize that programs that involve the whole school integrated into the school day tend to show more success than after-school programs. Examples of ASE programs developed in a school context are listed below (Table 11.3).

The Emotion-Based Prevention Program (PBE) or Emotion Course is an intervention developed over 20 weeks through three components: activities coordinated by teachers in the school context; observation and meetings with teachers by a team of specialists; in addition to parent involvement with monthly meetings and weekly messages about the emotion classes (Izard et al., 2008a). In our context, this program was adapted to Brazilian Portuguese by Otta, Andrade, Lucci and Abreu and is in the process of being published. The PBE includes various methodologies such

Table 11.3 Example of ASE Programs in the school context

Program name	Authors	Objectives	Age range
Friends of Zip	Clarke et al. (2014)	Promote mental health and well-being through the improvement of social and emotional skills, such as self-regulation and stress-coping skills	5–8 years
I Can Problem Solve *(ICPS)*	Shure (2001)	Promote pro-social behavior and reduce aggressive behaviors	3–6 years
MindUp: Mindfulness Education Program	Schonert-Reichl and Lawlor (2010)	Promote positive emotions, self-regulation, and goal setting	9–12 years
Intervention Program for the Promotion of Self-Regulation—PIPA	Dias and collaborators (2015)	Promote self-regulation skills with a special focus on emotion regulation.	3–5 years
Emotion-Based Prevention Program (PBE) or Emotion Course *(Emotion Course)*)	Izard et al. (2008a)	Foster the development of socio-emotional skills, reduce behavior problems, as well as potential precursors of psychopathologies in children, encouraging children to learn through emotional experiences	3–5 years
Promoting Alternative Thinking Strategies *(PATHS)*	Domitrovich et al., 2007	Promote social and emotional competence and reduce behavior problems	3–10 years
Child Regulation Therapy (TRI)—Preventive	Caminha and Caminha (n.d.)	Develop ASE through psychoeducation about emotions and the stimulation of emotional regulation through playful methodologies	5 and 6 years 8–11 years

as puppet play, storytelling, conversation circles, inductive dialogue, and hold tight technique (Hold Tight). Research conducted with the PBE with 191 children aged 3–5 years from low-income families in the United States showed that the children participating in this program improved their understanding and regulation of emotions. There was a decrease in emotional lability and negativity, aggressive, anxious and depressive behaviors, and negative expression of emotions (Izard et al., 2008a). The frequency of children with borderline or clinical scores for aggressive or anxious behaviors reduced in the group participating in the intervention, demonstrating that the PBE played a significant role in mental health prevention (Izard et al., 2008a).

Zippy's Friends is a program taught by teachers in a classroom context; it is based on the stories of the character Zippy in activities organized in modules with specific themes and objectives (Clarke et al., 2014). International research points to improvement in self-regulation, motivation and social skills (Clarke et al., 2014). In national studies, positive results of the intervention were reported in terms of communication and expression of feelings (Kovács, 2005). However, no significant differences were found in groups that underwent the intervention to reduce behavioral problems (Gomes, 2015).

The TRI-Preventive Program has two versions, considering neurodevelopmental aspects (Caminha & Caminha, n.d.). The TRI-Preventive Early Childhood Education is developed in 10 sessions in groups of children by a trained facilitator and an assistant. The program includes lectures for parents, educators, and the community and pedagogical team training. The TRI-Preventive for Elementary Education aims to prevent mood disorders and develop resilience strategies, lasting 18 h. No studies were found on the efficacy of the Program.

New techniques have been incorporated into ASE programs, such as the *Mindfulness* used in the MindUp Program. The training of *Mindfulness* aims to provide an exercise of the experience of the present moment that includes contemplation techniques, awareness in the here and now, breathing techniques and the internal reflection of thoughts and feelings without judgment, influenced by the Buddhist tradition and the meditative state (Zelazo & Lyons, 2012) (Chapter 10 of Volume 2 of Neuropsychological Interventions for Children will cover this topic). Programs that focus on stimulating executive functions for the school context also have activities aimed at the development of social and emotional skills, with emphasis on self-regulation, for example, the program *Tools of the Mind* (Bodrova & Leong, 2001).

Rehabilitation of Social and Emotional Skills in Neurodevelopmental Disorders

In the context of rehabilitation, different neurodevelopmental disorders present difficulties in the social and emotional domain, such as Autism Spectrum Disorder (ASD) and Attention Deficit Hyperactivity Disorder (ADHD), anxiety and mood disorders, in addition to genetic syndromes, for example, Williams Syndrome (Bellini et al., 2007; Järvinen et al., 2013; Rocca et al., 2009; Nijmeijer et al., 2008).

Compared to children with typical development, children with ADHD have difficulty in social cognition, mainly in the recognition of complex emotions, empathy, assertiveness, self-regulation, and participation (Pereira, 2017). In ADHD, there is also reported greater difficulty in maintaining friendships, as well as an increased risk for the development of psychiatric disorders (Nijmeijer et al., 2008). Another clinical condition that has been the focus of studies is Bipolar Mood Disorder (BMD), which may present difficulties in recognizing emotions in adult and child faces, as well as in judging the intensity of an emotional expression, which tend to be described as of lesser intensity (Rocca et al., 2009).

Difficulty in identifying and processing emotional information and various domains of social skills are widely portrayed in individuals with ASD. This population presents a shorter fixation time on the human face, especially in the eye region, compared to individuals with typical development and have significant impairments in recognizing basic emotions of fear, anger, disgust, and surprise. (Dalton et al., 2005; Klin et al., 2002). Generally, people with ASD have difficulties communicating, processing and integrating information from the environment, establishing and maintaining social relationships, interacting and participating in activities in new environments (Bellini et al., 2007), and global deficits in language in prosody, semantics, and pragmatics. There are also failures in the theory of mind, the ability to infer other people's mental and emotional states and beliefs. Social difficulties in ASD may include difficulties understanding the figurative use of language, ironies, jokes, and hidden intentions.

Intervention programs for children with ASD studied by McConnell (2002) were systematized from the following taxonomy:

(a) *Environmental modification* involves modifications in the physical and social environment to promote social interactions between children with ASD and their peers.
(b) *Specific interventions for children* involve the direct instruction of target social behaviors, such as initiation and appropriate response to context.
(c) *Interventions focusing on indirect skills* involve the training of skills not directly related to social skills; that is, it focuses on training related skills, such as playful behavior and language.
(d) *Peer-mediated interventions* involve the engagement of peers with typical development to respond and contribute to the direction and establishment of social behaviors of children with ASD.
(e) *Comprehensive interventions* involve social skills that combine two or more of the abovementioned intervention categories.

A meta-analysis reviewed 55 studies that investigated the effectiveness of school-based socio-emotional skills training programs for children and adolescents with ASD (Bellini et al., 2007). The results indicated that the effects were small for children with ASD, with low generalization; despite this, moderate effects of maintenance were observed and suggested gains from the social skills intervention after the end of the intervention. The interventions that showed the greatest effect were those carried out in the classroom, which produced intensification of the intervention, greater maintenance, and generalization of effects, compared to interventions that involved removing the child from the classroom (Bellini et al., 2007).

An example of a rehabilitation program for children with ASD is the animated series *The Transporters*, which consists of stories of cars with faces and facial expressions to train emotional understanding skills (Golan et al., 2010). The animated series was based on Baron-Cohen's hyper-systematization theory, which advocated that vehicles that use physical laws and are highly predictable in their movement (like rail vehicles that move back and forth) are preferred by children with ASD instead of vehicles like planes or cars whose movement varies greatly (Golan et al., 2010). The animation consists of 8 characters that are vehicles, with 15 episodes of 5 min each, so that each one focuses on a key emotion, such as joy, sadness, anger, fear, disgust, surprise, envy, shame, pride, among others. Throughout the episodes, the characters who are the means of transport with faces of real actors' emotional expressions present social interactions, thus creating a friendly and attractive environment for children with ASD (Golan et al., 2010). American and

Chinese children with ASD aged 4–7 who participated in the intervention *The Transporters* significantly improved in measures of emotional understanding (Golan et al., 2010; Yan et al., 2018).

Bauminger (2007) evaluated the effectiveness of multimodal cognitive-behavioral intervention and social skills training for a group of high-functioning pre-adolescents with autism. The ecological cognitive-behavioral intervention encompasses teaching interpersonal problem-solving based on short social vignettes that stimulate the discussion of essential social skills and using affective education and cognitive reconstruction using cartoon figures (Gray 1998, cited by Bauminger, 2007). Interaction between children was worked on through participation in cooperative social group activities and role-playing with same-age children. The social skills intervention focused on five topics:

(a) Instruction on the concept of group, group activities, and coexistence rules such as listening and respecting speaking turns
(b) Affective education involving verbal and non-verbal socio-emotional understanding and a greater understanding of complex emotions and their markers
(c) Group conversation skills
(d) Cooperation competencies, knowing the definition of cooperation and of shared interactive activity, mutual planning, and focus on pro-social skills for effective cooperation, such as commitment, encouragement, and comfort
(e) Understanding of sentences and uses of double entendre messages, recognizing cynicism or irony

Results indicated that there was a direct improvement in measures of social cognition and improvements in social relations, mainly social interactions and cooperation at the group level. No improvements were seen in dyads and social interactions during school recess.

Cognitive Behavioral Therapy (CBT) with children and adolescents has offered systematic resources for this age group to address the daily situations and actions experienced daily that can generate negative feelings associated with automatic thoughts (Petersen & Wainer, 2011). The clinical TRI (Caminha & Caminha, n.d.), like the preventive one (Caminha et al., 2015), proposes to work on the basic components of CBT (Emotion-Thought-Behavior) through adapted language using metaphors being: T—Work your emotions, R—Recycle your thoughts, and I—Innovate your behaviors). The TRI clinical protocol uses three technological instruments: the "Emotion Deck," the "Thought Deck," and the "Behavior Deck" (Caminha & Caminha, 2007, 2012, 2013), which have a playful and simple language for strategies of emotional self-regulation, empathy, understanding of emotions and thoughts.

New perspectives in neuropsychological rehabilitation have been made possible by technological advancement (Martin et al., 2014). Non-invasive neuromodulatory techniques have shown promising results for the promotion of social neuroplasticity, that is, the modulation of the functional and structural substrates of the nervous system associated with social and emotional skills aiming at healthy social interactions (Boggio et al., 2015; Malloy-Diniz et al., 2010) (Chapter 14 of Volume 2 of

Neuropsychological Interventions for Children will address this theme). At the same time, interventions with various methodologies, specifically with music, have also pointed to perspectives for rehabilitating socio-emotional skills in clinical populations. Studies conducted with children and adolescents with Williams Syndrome indicate that associating musical stimuli with affective valence to visual stimuli can enhance the understanding of facial emotions (Lense et al., 2014). At the same time, music relates to limbic and paralimbic brain structures, related to the generation, maintenance, termination, and modulation of emotions, being possible resources for treating affective disorders (Koelsch, 2009).

In the clinical context, various strategies are used to promote and develop social and emotional skills. The most commonly used strategies involve working from the recognition, naming, and identification of emotions in everyday contexts and situations as well as ER itself. In addition, it is necessary to promote psychoeducational activities to train social skills such as empathy, knowing how to put oneself in the other's perspective, assertiveness, and understanding one's own feelings and those of others. Breathing has also been used in various programs and techniques as an immediate means of regulating bodily arousal, especially in stronger emotions such as feelings of anger, injustice, and great dissatisfaction, such as the turtle technique, the hug technique, Stop and Think, Count to 10 and mindfulness training. *Mindfulness.* It is also important to provide means for the family to engage in rehabilitation with more ecological activities, and the professional should include specific activities to be worked on in non-clinical environments. Table 11.4 summarizes tips and strategies that can be used both in the clinical context and in the school and home context.

Final Considerations

Through a conceptual and empirical contextualization, this chapter sought to present programs and methodologies for stimulating and rehabilitating social and emotional skills in childhood. The presented research emphasizes the importance of interventions in socio-emotional skills for the promotion, prevention, treatment, and rehabilitation of health problems in children and adolescents. There is a significant gap and a need to strengthen this field within the scope of neuropsychology.

In the context of rehabilitation, programs and techniques based on evidence emphasizing understanding emotions, greater awareness about one's own mental states and feelings, as well as psychoeducational techniques and self-regulation strategies, stand out. New perspectives on neuromodulation technology are pointed out as promising. In stimulation, evidence corroborates that early interventions are necessary and especially effective, highlighting the important contribution that legislators, public managers, educators, and the general community can make to the healthy development of children by supporting the implementation of social and emotional learning programs in schools.

Table 11.4 Strategies for stimulating socio-emotional skills in various contexts

	School and home contexts	Clinical context
Understanding of Emotions	Pretend play, especially when needing to perform different roles that require different socio-emotional attitudes such as being a mother, or being a teacher or helping a friend who is sad. Dramatization and storytelling using dialogues and reflections that help children understand the emotions of characters. Use everyday social situations in which children are involved to help them identify and name their emotions and the emotions of their peers and/or adults. For example: "You are sad because you lost the doll you liked." Talk about what you are thinking, explore everyone's opinion and that people can feel and think differently. Play about the causes and consequences of emotions.	Games and activities that allow the naming of emotions. For example, use visual stimuli with images of facial emotions to be named. Games and activities associating social situations with emotional expressions through verbal labeling or facial expressions of emotions. Use of psychotherapeutic techniques that allow the child to understand their emotions and those of their social peers. Use of resources such as stories with emotional content and books that emphasize the expression, causes, and consequences of emotions. Dramatization of emotional situations. Psychoeducation systematically teaches and demonstrates the different emotions, involved situations, and their functions in social terms.
	Tips for dramatizing with emotions: Deck of emotions.	
Emotion regulation	When the child goes through a stressful situation, offer comfort and encourage them to talk about their feelings. Provide models of emotional self-regulation such as thinking in other ways, talking to someone, or doing an activity they enjoy. It is important to avoid suppressing intense emotions by saying, "You can't cry" or "I've already told you that you can't get angry or irritated." Instead, promote the identification of the emotion and think about ways to deal with it. Use everyday social situations to promote emotion regulation. Encourage children to verbalize their perceptions and emotions and communicate the reason for the conflict promotes the use of language to resolve it.	Emotion regulation techniques: Preschoolers: Turtle technique Hug technique School age onward: Stop and Think, traffic light analogy: (1) Stop at red: breathe or take time to calm down, count to 10; (2) Think at yellow: understand what is happening and think about how you can solve it; (3) Act at green: choose one of the actions you thought of to put into practice. Cognitive restructuring: reassess the situations experienced and the associated feelings.

(continued)

Table 11.4 (continued)

	School and home contexts	Clinical context
	For example, during a conflict between peers, you can ask the students how they are feeling and thinking and how they could resolve that conflict more assertively. Talk about the emotion at the time of occurrence in the child: "When we get very angry, we don't need to hit. Let's do something else to try to feel better. What can you do?" If any student is experiencing a very intense emotion, considering a certain situation, try to help them calm down, and use breathing techniques and emotion regulation strategies discussed in this chapter. If necessary, the teacher can mediate the dialogue between the children, promoting assertive expression and respect for the alternation of speaking turns. Encourage children to talk about what happened, helping them to name what they felt and reflect on their behavior. In group situations, in the face of various activities, such as, for example, games and competitive games, questions can be asked about how the members of the groups are feeling, allowing the validation of their emotions.	Provide models of pro-social behaviors to regulate negative emotions such as breathing, counting to 10, doing an activity pleasurable or energetic, and withdrawing from the situation. Visualization techniques to encourage self-regulation. *Mindfulness:* contemplation activities, awareness in the here and now, and breathing practices to promote focus on what is being done.
Empathy	Games that require putting oneself in the other's place. Parents can encourage their children to understand that their tastes and feelings differ from those of others. Pretend Play Games	The therapist can provide *scripts* or narratives to exemplify effective forms of empathy (for example, What would you do if your friend were sad? You could talk to him and hug him). In addition, it can generate reflection on the stories and narratives in regard to the attitude of the characters. In moments of free play, it can provide moments that require putting oneself in the place of others to decide what to do.

References

Arango, M. I. R. (2007). Regulación emocional y competência social em la infância. *Diversitas: Perspectivas em Psicologia, 3*(2), 349–363.

Bauminger, N. (2007). Brief report: Group social-multimodal intervention for HFASD. *Journal of Autism and Developmental Disorders, 37*(8), 1605–1615. https://doi.org/10.1007/s10803-006-0246-3

Bellini, S., Peters, J. K., Benner, L., & Hopf, A. (2007). A meta-analysis of school-based social skills interventions for children with autism spectrum disorders. *Remedial and Special Education, 28*(3), 153–162. https://doi.org/10.1177/07419325070280030401

Bennett, D. S., Bendersky, M., & Lewis, M. (2005). Antecedents of emotion knowledge: Predictors of individual differences in young children. *Cognition & Emotion, 19*(3), 375–396. https://doi.org/10.1080/02699930441000201

Bergamasco, N. H. P. (1997). Expressão Facial Como Acesso À Consciência do Recém-Nascido. *Psicologia USP, 8*(2), 275–286. https://doi.org/10.1590/S0103-65641997000200013

Bodrova, E., & Leong, D. J. (2001). *Tools of the mind: A case study of implementing the Vygotskian approach in American early childhood and primary classrooms.* International Bureau of Education, UNESCO.

Boggio, P. S., Asthana, M. K., Costa, T. L., Valasek, C. A., & Osorio, A. A. (2015). Promoting social plasticity in developmental disorders with non-invasive brain stimulation techniques. *Frontiers in Neuroscience, 9*, 294. https://doi.org/10.3389/fnins.2015.00294

Bosacki,S.L.,&Moore,C.(2004).Preschoolers' understandingofsimpleandcomplexemotions:Links with gender and language. *Sex Roles*. https://doi.org/10.1023/B:SERS.0000027568.26966.27

Bussab, V. S. R., & Ribeiro, F. L. (1998). Biologicamente cultural. Psicologia: reflexões (im)pertinentes, 175–193.

Caminha, R. M., & Caminha, M. G. (2007). *Baralho das emoções: acessando a criança no trabalho clínico*. Sinopsys Editora.

Caminha, R. M., & Caminha, M. G. (2012). *Baralho dos pensamentos: reciclando ideias, promovendo consciência*. Sinopsys Editora.

Caminha, R. M., & Caminha, M. G. (2013). *Baralho dos comportamentos: efeito bumerangue*. Sinopsys Editora.

Caminha, R. M. , & Caminha, M. G. (n.d.). Terapia de Regulação Infantil – TRI.

Caminha, M. G., Caminha, R. M., & Justo, A. R. (2015). Trabalho de Reciclagem Infantil – Preventivo (TRI-P): Aplicação em grupo de escolares. In C. B. Neufeld (Ed.), *Terapia Cognitivo-Comportamental em grupo para crianças e adolescentes*. Artmed.

Clarke, A. M., Bunting, B., & Barry, M. M. (2014). Evaluating the implementation of a school-based emotional well-being programme: A cluster randomized controlled trial of Zippy's Friends for children in disadvantaged primary schools. *Health Education Research., 29*(5), 786–798. https://doi.org/10.1093/her/cyu047

Coll, C., Marchesi, A., & Palácios, J. (2004). *Desenvolvimento psicológico e educação: psicologia evolutiva*. Artmed.

Dalton, K. M., Nacewicz, B. M., Johnstone, T., Schaefer, H. S., & Gernsbacher, M. A. (2005). Gaze fixation and the neural circuitry of face processing in autism. *Nature Neuroscience, 8*, 519–526.

Denham, S. A. (1998). *Emotional development in young children*. The Guilford.

Denham, S. a., Caverly, S., Schmidt, M., Blair, K., DeMulder, E., Caal, S., Hideko, H., & Mason, T. (2002). Preschool understanding of emotions: Contributions to classroom anger and aggression. *Journal of Child Psychology and Psychiatry, and Allied Disciplines, 43*(7), 901–916. https://doi.org/10.1111/1469-7610.00139

Denham, S. a., Bassett, H. H., Mincic, M., Kalb, S., Way, E., Wyatt, T., & Segal, Y. (2012). Social-emotional learning profiles of preschoolers' early school success: A person-centered approach. *Learning and Individual Differences, 22*(2), 178–189. https://doi.org/10.1016/j.lindif.2011.05.001

Dias, N. M., & Seabra, A. G. (2013). *Programa de Intervenção em Autorregulação e Funções Executivas – PIAFEx*. Memnon.
Dias, N. M., Mecca, T. P., León, C. R., Zauza, G., Muniz, M., & Seabra, A. G. (2015). Programa de Intervenção para Promoção de Autorregulação – PIPA.
Domitrovich, C. E., Cortes, R. C., & Greenberg, M. T. (2007). Improving young children's social and emotional competence: A randomized trial of the preschool "PATHS" curriculum. *The Journal of Primary Prevention, 28*(2), 67–91. https://doi.org/10.1007/s10935-007-0081-0
Durlak, J. A., & Wells, A. M. (1997). Primary prevention mental health programs for children and adolescents. *American Journal of Community Psychology, 25*(2), 115–152.
Durlak, J. A., Weissberg, R. P., Dymnicki, A. B., Taylor, R. D., & Schellinger, K. B. (2011). The impact of enhancing students' social and emotional learning: A meta-analysis of school-based universal interventions. *Child Development, 82*(1), 405–432. https://doi.org/10.1111/j.1467-8624.2010.01564.x
Eisenberg, N., Fabes, R. A., Murphy, B., Karbon, M., Maszk, P., Smith, M., & Suh, K. (1994). The relations of emotionality and regulation to dispositional and situational empathy-related responding. *Journal of Personality and Social Psychology, 66*(4), 776.
Eisenberg, N., Spinrad, T. L., & Eggum, N. D. (2010). Emotion-related self-regulation and its relation to children's maladjustment. *Annual Review of Clinical Psychology, 6*, 495–525. https://doi.org/10.1146/annurev.clinpsy.121208.131208
Fernandéz- Abascal, E. G., Rodríguez, B. G., Sanchez, M. P. J., Díaz, M. D. M., & Sánchez, F. J. D. (2010). *Psicologia de la emoción*. Editorial Ramón Areces.
Fredrickson, B. L., & Levenson, R. W. (1998). Positive emotions speed recovery from the cardiovascular sequelae of negative emotions. *Cognition & Emotion, 12*, 191–220.
Frey, K. S., Nolen, S. B., Van Schoiack Edstrom, L., & Hirschstein, M. K. (2005). Effects of a school-based social–emotional competence program: Linking children's goals, attributions, and behavior. *Journal of Applied Developmental Psychology, 26*(2), 171–200. https://doi.org/10.1016/j.appdev.2004.12.002
Golan, O., Ashwin, E., Granader, Y., McClintock, S., Day, K., Leggett, V., & Baron-Cohen, S. (2010). Enhancing emotion recognition in children with autism spectrum conditions: An intervention using animated vehicles with real emotional faces. *Journal of Autism and Developmental Disorders, 40*(3), 269–279. https://doi.org/10.1007/s10803-009-0862-9
Gomes, R. T. M. (2015). Avaliação do Impacto de um Programa de Educação Emocional em sala de aula na percepção de professores, pais e alunos: Amigos do Zippy. Universidade Federal de São Paulo (Dissertação de Mestrado). https://doi.org/10.1007/s13398-014-0173-7.2
Gross, J. J. (2007). *Handbook of emotion regulation*. Guilford Press.
Izard, C. E. (2001). Emotional intelligence or adaptive emotions? *Emotion, 1*(3), 249–257. https://doi.org/10.1037//1528-3542.1.3.249
Izard, C. E. (2002). Translating emotion theory and research into preventive interventions. *Psychological Bulletin, 128*(5), 796–824. https://doi.org/10.1037//0033-2909.128.5.796
Izard, C. E. (2004). Emotions theory for teachers: Concepts and principle for the emotions course. Adaptação brasileira, Otta, E., Andrade, N. C., Lucci, T. K., & Abreu, N. (no prelo).
Izard, C. E. (2009). Emotion theory and research: Highlights, unanswered questions, and emerging issues. *Annual Review of Psychology, 60*, 1–25. https://doi.org/10.1146/annurev.psych.60.110707.163539.Emotion
Izard, C. E., Fine, S., Mostow, A., Trentacosta, C., & Campbell, J. (2002). Emotion processes in normal and abnormal development and preventive intervention. *Development and Psychopathology, 14*(4), 761–787. https://doi.org/10.1017/S0954579408000175. Retrieved from http://www.ncbi.nlm.nih.gov/pubmed/12549703, 20(1), 369–397
Izard, C. E., King, K. A., Trentacosta, C. J., Morgan, J. K., Laurenceau, J.-P., Krauthamer-Ewing, E. S., & Finlon, K. J. (2008a). Accelerating the development of emotion competence in Head Start children: Effects on adaptive and maladaptive behavior. *Development and Psychopathology, 20*(1), 369–397. https://doi.org/10.1017/S0954579408000175

Izard, C. E., Stark, K., Trentacosta, C., & Schultz, D. (2008b). Beyond emotion regulation: Emotion utilization and adaptive functioning. *Child Development Perspectives, 2*(3), 156–163. https://doi.org/10.1111/j.1750-8606.2008.00058.x

Järvinen, A., Korenberg, J. R., & Bellugi, U. (2013). The social phenotype of Williams syndrome. *Current Opinion in Neurobiology, 23*(3), 414–422. https://doi.org/10.1016/j.conb.2012.12.006

Klin, A., Jones, W., Schultz, R., Volkmar, F., & Cohen, D. (2002). Visual fixation patterns during viewing of naturalistic social situations as predictors of social competence in individuals with autism. *Archives of General Psychiatry, 59*, 809–816.

Koelsch, S. (2009). A neuroscientific perspective on music therapy. *Annals of the New York Academy of Sciences, 1169*(1), 374–384. https://doi.org/10.1111/j.1749-6632.2009.04592.x

Kovács, M. J. (2005). Avaliação do programa Amigos do Zippy.

Kraag, G., Zeegers, M. P., Kok, G., Hosman, C., & Abu-Saad, H. H. (2006). School programs targeting stress management in children and adolescents: A meta-analysis. *Journal of School Psychology, 44*(6), 449–472. https://doi.org/10.1016/j.jsp.2006.07.001

Lemerise, E. A., & Arsenio, W. F. (2000). An integrated model of emotion processes and cognition in social information processing. *Child Development, 71*, 107–118.

Lense, M. D., Gordon, R. L., Key, A. P. F., & Dykens, E. M. (2014). Neural correlates of cross-modal affective priming by music in Williams syndrome. *Social Cognitive and Affective Neuroscience, 9*(4), 529–537. https://doi.org/10.1093/scan/nst017

Liao, Z., Li, Y., & Su, Y. (2014). Emotion understanding and reconciliation in overt and relational conflict scenarios among preschoolers. *International Journal of Behavioral Development, 38*(5), 111–117. https://doi.org/10.1177/0165025413512064

Liotti, M., & Panksepp, J. (2004). On the neural nature of human emotions and implications for biological psychiatry. In J. Panksepp (Ed.), *Textbook of biological psychiatry* (pp. 33–74). Wiley.

Malloy-Diniz, L. F., Fuentes, D., Mattos, P., & Abreu, N. (2010). *Avaliação Neuropsicológica*. Artmed.

Martin, D. M., Liu, R., Alonzo, A., Green, M., & Loo, C. K. (2014). Use of transcranial direct current stimulation (tDCS) to enhance cognitive training: Effect of timing of stimulation. *Experimental Brain Research, 232*(10), 3345–3351.

McConnell, S. (2002). Interventions to facilitate social interaction for young children with autism: Review of available research and recommendations for educational intervention and future research. *Journal of Autism and Developmental Disorders, 32*(5), 351–372. https://doi.org/10.1023/A:1020537805154

Miller, A. L., Hospital, E. P. B., Seifer, R., Eguia, M., Gouley, K. K., Seifer, R., Zakriski, A., Eguia, M., & Vergnani, M. (2005). Emotion knowledge skills in low-income elementary school children: Associations with social status and peer experiences. *Social Development, 14*(4), 637–651. https://doi.org/10.1111/j.1467-9507.2005.00321.x

Morgan, J. K., Izard, C. E., & King, K. A. (2010). Construct validity of the emotion matching task: Preliminary evidence for convergent and criterion validity of a new emotion knowledge measure for young children. *Social Development, 19*(1), 52–70. https://doi.org/10.1111/j.1467-9507.2008.00529.x

Nijmeijer, J. S., Minderaa, R. B., Buitelaar, J. K., Mulligan, A., Hartman, C. A., & Hoekstra, P. J. (2008). Attention-deficit/hyperactivity disorder and social dysfunctioning. *Clinical Psychology Review, 28*(4), 692–708. https://doi.org/10.1016/j.cpr.2007.10.003

Pereira, C. F. (2017). Funções Executivas e Cognição Social em crianças com Transtorno do Déficit de Atenção e Hiperatividade. Dissertação (Dissertação de Mestrado). Universidade Federal de Campinas, Faculdade de Ciências Médicas.

Peretz, I. (2009). Towards a neurobiology of musical emotion. In *Handbook of music and emotion: Theory, research, applications* (pp. 99–126). Oxford University Press.

Petersen, C. S., & Wainer, R. (2011). *Terapias Cognitivo-comportamentais para crianças e adolescentes*. Artmed.

Phan, K. L., Wager, T., Taylor, S. F., & Liberzon, I. (2002). Functional neuroanatomy of emotion: A meta-analysis of emotion activation studies in PET and fMRI. *NeuroImage, 16*(2), 331–348. https://doi.org/10.1006/nimg.2002.1087

Puerta, M. L. S., Valerio, A., & Bernal, M. G. (2016). *Taking stock of programs to develop socioemotional skills: A systematic review of program evidence*. World Bank. https://doi.org/10.1596/978-1-4648-0872-2

Ribeiro, F. L., Bussab, V. L., & Otta, E. (2004). De colo em colo, de berço em berço. In *O bebê do século XXI e a psicologia em desenvolvimento*. Casa do Psicólogo.

Rocca, C. C. A., Heuvel, E. D., Caetano, S. C., & Lafer, B. (2009). Facial emotion recognition in bipolar disorder: A critical review. *Revista Brasileira de Psiquiatria, 31*(2), 171–180.

Schonert-Reichl, K. A., & Lawlor, M. S. (2010). The effects of a mindfulness-based education program on pre- and early adolescents' well-being and social and emotional competence. *Mindfulness*. https://doi.org/10.1007/s12671-010-0011-8

Schultz, D., Izard, C., Ackerman, B. P., Youngstrom, E. A., & Hall, W. (2001). Emotion knowledge in economically disadvantaged children: Self-regulatory antecedents and relations to social difficulties and withdrawal. *Development and Psychopathology, 13*(1), 53–67.

Shure, M. B. (2001). I can problem solve (ICPS): An interpersonal cognitive problem solving program for children. *Residential Treatment for Children & Youth, 18*(3), 3–14.

Sprung, M., Münch, H. M., Harris, P. L., Ebesutani, C., & Hofmann, S. G. (2015). Children's emotion understanding: A meta-analysis of training studies. *Developmental Review, 37*, 41–65. https://doi.org/10.1016/j.dr.2015.05.001

Trentacosta, C. J., & Fine, S. E. (2010). Emotion knowledge, social competence, and behavior problems in childhood and adolescence: A meta-analytic review. *Social Development, 19*, 1–29. https://doi.org/10.1111/J.1467-9507.2009.00543.X

Trentacosta, C. J., & Izard, C. E. (2007). Kindergarten children's emotion competence as a predictor of their academic competence in first grade. *Emotion, 7*(1), 77–88. https://doi.org/10.1037/1528-3542.7.1.77

Yan, Y., Liu, C., Ye, L., & Liu, Y. (2018). Using animated vehicles with real emotional faces to improve emotion recognition in Chinese children with autism spectrum disorder. *PLoS ONE, 13*(7), 1–6. https://doi.org/10.1371/journal.pone.0200375

Zelazo, P. D., & Lyons, K. E. (2012). The potential benefits of mindfulness training in early childhood: A developmental social cognitive neuroscience perspective. *Child Development Perspectives, 6*(2), 154–160. https://doi.org/10.1111/j.1750-8606.2012.00241.x

Chapter 12
Intervention in Mathematical Skills: Number Sense

Luciana Vellinho Corso, Helena Vellinho Corso, and Jerusa Fumagalli de Salles

Number sense, a concept encompassing a set of skills vital for competence in mathematics, is a complex phenomenon. Its development requires a set of individual, environmental, and school conditions, acting in an integrated manner.

In some Latin American countries, including Brazil, low performance levels, evidenced by school censuses (OECD, 2016), reveal lags in the area of Mathematics from very early in the school trajectory of many students, creating gaps that can extend throughout the learner's life. Naturally, the impact of such a situation brings disastrous consequences for the individual and society as a whole: high rates of school dropout, lower levels of higher education, high rates of unemployment and underemployment, as well as high levels of psychological suffering, low esteem, and anxiety (Piccolo et al., 2017). Therefore, preventive neuropsychological intervention (capable of identifying students at risk of developing learning problems) and remedial (capable of addressing the obstacles that prevent certain learning) are coping strategies for the difficult situation mentioned. Similarly, different classroom approaches, focusing on acquiring and developing mathematical skills, play a fundamental role in preventing future difficulties and in the specific interventions necessary throughout the student's school journey.

The significant difficulty in learning mathematics is highlighted by DSM 5 (Diagnostic and Statistical Manual of Mental Disorders) as a Specific Learning Disorder, with impairment in Mathematics in one or more of the following aspects: number sense, memorization of arithmetic facts, accuracy or fluency of calculation and/or accuracy in mathematical reasoning (American Psychiatric Association [APA], 2014).

L. V. Corso · H. V. Corso (✉) · J. F. de Salles
Universidade Federal do Rio Grande do Sul, Porto Alegre, Brazil
e-mail: l.corso@terra.com.br; hvcorso@gmail.com; jerusafsalles@gmail.com

C. O. Cardoso, N. M. Dias (eds.), *Neuropsychological Interventions for Children - Volume 1*, https://doi.org/10.1007/978-3-031-53586-4_12

Number Sense

Number sense comprises a complex and multifaceted construct that enables the use of mathematical skills to face daily needs (Greeno, 1991). Such a field of study is characterized by conceptual controversies regarding the best way to conceptualize, assess, and intervene in number sense (Corso & Dorneles, 2010). Researchers in the field evidence consensus in regard to the following aspects: a well-developed numerical sense is at the base of competence in mathematics (Passolunghi & Lanfranchi, 2012) and, therefore, such a construct is a good initial detector of difficulties in arithmetic (Jordan et al., 2010; Passolunghi & Lanfranchi, 2012). Alongside this, a weakness in numerical sense is one of the characteristics that accompanies students with difficulties in mathematics (Geary, 2011), and problems with numerical sense can be identified early in Early Childhood Education (Jordan et al., 2010; Passolunghi & Lanfranchi, 2012). Findings of this type influence investigations on preventive and remedial intervention in this area (Jordan et al., 2010; Kuhn & Holling, 2014).

The lack of consensus among researchers when the purpose is to define numerical sense is striking. While some highlight in their definitions the conceptual, abstract part of numerical processing, such as the ability to represent and mentally manipulate numbers and quantities (Gersten et al., 2005), fluency and flexibility with numbers and understanding the meaning of numbers and ideas related to them (Gersten & Chard, 1999), other researchers emphasize performance that is facilitated by a conceptual understanding of number, such as counting ability, number identification, number knowledge, estimation, the concept of measure, and the ability to perform mental operations with numbers (Jordan et al., 2010). It seems to us that both ways of defining numerical sense can be seen as complementary since an abstract understanding of numerical processing is necessary to succeed in understanding and executing tasks involving numbers, numerical relations, and quantities (Corso, 2018). Therefore, the understanding of numerical sense that characterizes this chapter is that it is a general construct that encompasses a very broad set of concepts, which the student develops gradually from their interactions with the social environment. Numerical sense is a way of interacting with numbers, with their various uses and interpretations, enabling the individual to deal with daily situations that include quantifications and the development of efficient strategies (including mental calculation and estimation) to deal with numerical problems (Corso & Dorneles, 2010).

Research shows that number sense arises from a biological apparatus that allows the subject to pay attention to numerosity (Dehaene, 2001). In addition, social experiences play a fundamental role in the construction of numerical knowledge. The innate capacity for quantitative skills (implicit understanding of numerosity, ordinality, counting, and simple arithmetic) develops gradually over the preschool years, along with the structuring of language, even without formal education. From then on, quantitative skills become secondary, as they are determined by the education system of the culture in which they are inserted (Silva et al., 2015a, b). Therefore, numerical sense has an innate base that needs to be built and developed through interactions with the social environment.

Numerical processing and arithmetic operations occur based on three systems of mental representation, which characterize the theoretical model of the triple code (Dehaene & Cohen, 1995). This model proposes that numbers are processed in three different but interconnected circuits: one circuit responsible for the perception of magnitude, another for the visual representation of numerical symbols (Arabic numerals: 2, 4, 5) and the third responsible for the verbal representation of numbers (*two, four, five*). The multiple components of the model can be engaged in different combinations (Haase et al., 2015). Thus, an underdeveloped numerical sense occurs due to an immature representation and/or processing of numbers (Geary, 2011), which may encompass one or more of the mentioned circuits, causing lags in understanding and flexibility in their use and leading to problems for the development of skills such as counting, performing operations, estimates, and mental calculation, aspects that are fundamental for the development of fluency in mathematics (Corso & Dorneles, 2010; Geary, 2011).

Number sense is evaluated through a series of tasks that include a set of skills presumed to compose the construct: counting, counting principles, counting procedures and strategies, numerical sequence, basic facts of verbal and non-verbal addition and subtraction, math problems, understanding of magnitude, and estimation. The literature highlights the Number Knowledge Test by Okamoto and Case (1996) and the *Number Sense Brief* by Jordan et al. (2010) as good measures of number sense (Baker et al., 2002). These are informal research tasks, not standardized or normed. Still, they allow for the evaluation of the process and allow the examiner to make a detailed reading of the errors evidenced by the subject, which serves as an important source of information for the intervention process. The Battery of Neuropsychological Tests for Numerical Processing and Calculation in Children, revised version, known as Zareki-R (Silva et al., 2015b), is another internationally recognized instrument and aims to identify and specify, through 12 tasks, the profile of mathematical skills related to calculation and number processing in children.

It is important to remember that the development of number sense relies on specific domain competencies (basic numerical competencies) and general cognitive competencies, and both support the learning of mathematics (Corso & Dorneles, 2013). Counting (Stock et al., 2009), arithmetic calculation (Tolar et al., 2016), numerical magnitude comparison (De Smedt & Gilmore, 2011), and solving math problems (Fuchs et al., 2008) are some specific domain competencies that are strongly related to mathematical performance. As for general domain competencies, working memory (WM) (Corso & Dorneles, 2012; Geary, 2011), phonological processing through phonological memory (Hecht et al., 2001) and processing speed (Bull & Johnston, 1997; Nelson & Powell, 2017), and visuospatial skills (Haase et al., 2012) are domains that show associations with number sense. WM, in its central executive, phonological, and visuospatial components, is pointed out as one of the functions most involved with arithmetic processes (Chen et al., 2018; Corso, 2018; Corso & Dorneles, 2015; Haase et al., 2012; Toll et al., 2011). Inhibition, updating (*updating*) and switching (*switching/shifting*) are signaled as executive functions that need to be efficient for good mathematical performance (Bull & Lee, 2014; Chen et al., 2018; Cragg et al., 2017).

Among the general domain competencies, WM has gained increasing prominence in the literature (Jordan et al., 2010; Passolunghi & Lanfranchi, 2012), with investigations of the associations between the different components of WM and performance in number sense. Among the components of WM, the central executive, with its distinct functions, has been the most studied. There is no consensus about the role that each function of the central executive plays in number sense. Some studies suggest that inhibition plays an important role in predicting performance in number sense (Kroesbergen et al., 2009). Still, such result was not verified in other investigations (e.g., Lee et al., 2012). The update function is most commonly pointed out as a predictor of number sense (Kroesbergen et al., 2009; Lee et al., 2012).

Friso-van den Bos et al. (2013) conducted a meta-analysis involving 15 studies with children aged 4–12 years. The studies included at least one measure of number sense and one or more of the functions of the central executive component of WM (update, inhibition, switching). The authors found an association between number sense and the functions of updating and inhibition, and updating showed the highest correlation with number sense. Similarly, Corso (2018) showed that, among the functions of the central executive, updating has the highest correlation with number sense. The author emphasizes that dealing with proposals encompassing counting, performing operations, estimates, and mental calculation (tasks that make up the Numerical Knowledge Test) requires the involvement of the WM's updating function. During counting, for example, in executing a simple arithmetic calculation, it is necessary to maintain and process intermediate results in WM until the final result of the calculation can be reached. The central executive component of WM seems to be in high demand. At the same time, students have not yet acquired an automatism related to many of the skills necessary to succeed in math (for example, the automatic retrieval of basic arithmetic facts), an automatism that, it is hoped, will be achieved as the student progresses in school. However, the transition from a more conscious monitoring of the student (using earlier counting strategies, for example) to an automatism in calculation goes through a process that, until it is more mature, will require a greater demand from WM.

Preventive and Remedial Intervention in Number Sense

Number sense proves to be susceptible to intervention through explicit teaching of the aspects of this construct or arithmetic concepts that are underdeveloped in the student (Corso & Dorneles, 2010). Appropriate intervention is beneficial at any time. However, early intervention can prevent the development of negative attitudes and anxiety towards math (Dowker, 2005).

Intervention proposals aim to increase/complexify learning experiences in number sense planned based on each learner's individual needs (neuropsychological profile). Because they have difficulties in this domain, learners do not interact meaningfully with contexts involving numbers (quantifying, relating and comparing), which naturally accentuates their initial difficulties.

Intervention programs with a preventive focus, offered to all children and not just those with difficulties in math, are highlighted in the international literature (Dowker, 2005). Proposals of this type include introducing activities and math games in the early childhood education curriculum and, in some cases, helping parents use educational materials at home with their children. Response to intervention (RTI) programs, as a support system, early detection and intervention, demonstrate the effectiveness of early interventions in students with low performance in different aspects of number sense (Bryant et al., 2011).

Interventions in number sense adopt different paths; some include only the numerical competencies that need to be enhanced in the student (counting, storage of arithmetic combinations, teaching shortcuts like decomposition strategy, commutativity principle) (Dyson et al., 2011). Others associate the teaching of general domain competencies, including, for example, intervention in working memory and processing speed (Kuhn & Holling, 2014). Proposals of this type reinforce the role of cognitive skills in math competence.

When planning interventions, some principles prove to be fundamental to ensure success (Fuchs et al., 2010, 2013), among which stand out: explicit instruction, organization of small and interactive groups, presentation of content gradually and sequentially instead of simultaneously, promotion of the practice of the taught content, and favoring student motivation in pursuit of their engagement in the proposal and regulation of attention to activities.

Research indicates that brief interventions focusing on basic numerical skills, administered by teachers, clinicians, or researchers, are effective. Aragon-Mendizábal et al. (2017) conducted an intervention focusing on classification, solving addition and subtraction problems, distribution, discrimination, and seriation. The study involved 156 preschool children with low arithmetic performance over 5 weeks, with three weekly meetings of 30–35 min. After the intervention, the children in the experimental group demonstrated better performance compared to the controls. In a relatively recent study, Assis (2018) developed a brief intervention involving four teaching sessions on counting principles with 136 first-grade students. The students in the experimental group demonstrated superior advances in counting ability compared to the students in the control group.

Dyson et al. (2011) developed an interventional study on numerical competencies with preschool children from low-income communities who are at risk of developing difficulties in mathematics. The children were divided into intervention groups (30-min sessions three times a week, totaling 24 sessions) and a control group (*business-as-usual*). The intervention group showed significantly better performance than the controls (immediate post-test) in measures of numerical competencies and general mathematics. The permanence of the children's acquisitions (progress) was evidenced 8 weeks after the intervention.

Compared to the control, significant gains in the experimental group were also shown in the intervention study by Bryant et al. (2011), which involved 204 first-grade students. The intervention consisted of 4 weekly 25-min sessions for 19 weeks and focused on different aspects of number sense: counting; number recognition; comparison and grouping of numbers; more or less relations; part-whole relations; numerical sequencing; making and counting tens and units; positional value; reading and writing numerals to represent base ten models; counting strategies and decomposition; and properties of addition.

The study by Praet and Desoete (2014) involved using computer games to improve arithmetic skills in 132 preschool children. The intervention took place over nine sessions of 25 min for 5 weeks. Two experimental groups (in counting and in magnitude comparison) and control were subjected to the intervention, and the results in arithmetic skills were more significant for the experimental groups. The effects of the intervention were observed up to 6 months after its completion.

The use of technologies, with the aim of offering and mediating learning situations that favor the creation of connections between conceptual and procedural knowledge, characterizes some intervention programs in number sense, such as computer games using specific mathematical content and skills, such as *Number Race*[1] (Wilson et al., 2006), available on the web, and *The Road to Mathematics* (Toll, 2013). Specific software also encourages spatial representation of numbers on the number line (Kucian et al., 2011).

A more recent trend in intervention research in number sense is the combination of interventions in general domain skills, such as MT, for example, with the specific sub-areas of mathematics in which the student shows delays (Melby-Lervag & Hulme, 2013). Interventions of this type can bring promising results. In this line of research, Kuhn and Holling (2014) compared the mathematical skills of students without difficulties in mathematics who received intervention in MT or in number sense from pre- to post-test. Both interventions led to improvement in the mathematical skills of the students compared to the control group. Another example of combined intervention was carried out in the study by Fuchs et al. (2013) with first-grade students at risk of developing problems in mathematics. The children received intervention in number knowledge, associated or not with intervention in processing speed (practices that reinforced quick responses to number facts and the efficient use of counting procedures). The students who received both interventions showed better results in simple and 2-digit arithmetic calculations compared to those who did not receive the intervention in processing speed.

Sperafico (2016) compared the effects of a combined intervention in arithmetic reasoning (addition and multiplication relations) and MT, applied to 46 students with Attention Deficit Hyperactivity Disorder (ADHD) with an intervention of the same duration only in MT. The students who received the combined intervention performed better in calculation and arithmetic reasoning than those who had intervention only in MT. Nunes et al. (2014) also present evidence of the positive effects of interventions specially designed to improve performance in mathematics through

[1] The *Number Race* : http://www.thenumberrace.com/nr/home.php

computer games with an emphasis on MT tasks. This work was carried out with deaf children.

Finally, the works presented show that interventions specifically planned to prevent and/or remedy difficulties with number sense, in its different aspects, present promising results. However, unfortunately, in many contexts and locations there is still a gap between research results and school and clinical practice, which ends up delaying the possibility of helping students with difficulties in this area. In addition, most of the intervention research cited is not available in Portuguese, and national studies on number sense are scarce. Therefore, there is an urgent need for investment in collaborative research. With advances in investigations, it is expected to fill the existing gaps in evaluation and intervention in number sense.

Number Sense and Educational Practices

As mentioned, an underdeveloped number sense is pointed out as one of the potential causes of learning problems in mathematics, and specific interventions in this area have shown promising results. Thus, it is worth reflecting on the impact of such results on school practices.

Unfortunately, the influences of studies on number sense on educational practices, in many contexts, like the Brazilian one, are slow. As a consequence, students with difficulties in mathematics are not understood in the classroom and do not receive teaching appropriate to their peculiarities (Dorneles & Haase, 2017). The emphasis of teaching continues to be on the repetition of calculation processes and memorization of formulas devoid of meaning for the student, to the detriment of teaching basic principles of number sense such as comparison of magnitude, ability to use the number line, and estimation. Little is done in relation to teaching counting strategies, decomposition, and memory retrieval that help the student acquire automaticity and confidence in mathematics (Corso & Assis, 2017).

Strengthening number sense favors the development of conceptual knowledge necessary for arithmetic resolution (counting experiences that allow the discovery of mathematical relationships). Similarly, it enables practice using more mature and efficient counting strategies. The contextualized practice of strategies works as a kind of scaffolding for developing strategies based on immediate memory retrieval. The retrieval of arithmetic facts from memory, in turn, plays an important role in developing more complex mathematical processes (*e.g.*, multi-digit calculation, problem-solving). Therefore, placing more emphasis on teaching this skill is important, especially for students struggling with math.

Another point to highlight in relation to teaching, in addition to the key aspects of number sense, is the need to consider students' cognitive possibilities, as these directly influence their learning. The way teaching is conducted will directly influence the effect of potential cognitive deficits on learning. For example, learning multiplication may be difficult for students who struggle to retrieve facts from memory if teaching is based purely on memorizing the times tables. But, on the contrary, if the teacher focuses on understanding basic facts and teaching action strategies on which the students can rely to compensate for their memory difficulty, then learning multiplication will not be a big problem for them. Even a student who is too slow to calculate will need the teaching of more mature and efficient counting strategies and procedures so that they do not need to rely too much on working memory (as happens when the procedure of counting all the parcels of the operation is used), overloading it and increasing the chance of error in the calculation (Corso & Dorneles, 2014).

It is clear, then, that the teaching of initial mathematics deserves double attention. A promising path is the constant exchanges between academic production and classroom practice. An example of this perspective is presented in the work of Nunes and collaborators (2005), *"Mathematics Education: Numbers and Numerical Operations."* The material presents a proposal for teaching initial mathematics from the perspective of evidence-based education. Planning teaching based on evidence suggests constant evaluation of the student's understanding of number, numbering system, additive reasoning, and quantitative reasoning, among other aspects. The work offers numerous problem situations that elicit the use of a variety of strategies by the student. In this way, this perspective contemplates not only the student's learning but also the teacher's learning process.

Following the same action proposal, the *Numeracy Corner* (Nunes & Moreno, 2002; Nunes, 2009), although in English, is easy to understand, contains a series of activities with illustrations of problem situations that involve arithmetic reasoning (additive composition, additive and multiplicative reasoning), and can be used for evaluation and/or intervention with the mediation of the teacher/clinician. The material was originally developed for work with deaf children but is also used with other groups of students and can be found at: http://www.education.ox.ac.uk/ndcs/Resources/teachersbook_exercises.pdf.

The same research group also offers online material composed of games, the Games Corner, aimed at intervention in numeracy, literacy, and working memory. The program develops metacognitive skills and automatic attention and can be accessed at http://www.education.ox.ac.uk/ndcs/index.php.

The *Dybuster Calcularis* (Santos, 2017) is a digital intervention for training mathematical skills in children and adolescents in Elementary School. The program comprises number processing, addition-subtraction and multiplication-division (http://www.calcularis.com.br). The student has the possibility to train skills such as estimation and *subtizing* (the ability to recognize and distinguish numerical sets with up to 3 or 4 stimuli without having to count them); numerical understanding (verbal, numerical, and analog); transcoding; number line; greater-less and numerical intervals. The pilot study by Käser et al. (2013) investigated the effect of using the *Calcularis* program on Swiss children with difficulties in mathematics who underwent 12 weeks of training. The results showed improvements in basic mathematical skills (estimation on the number line) and in arithmetic operations of addition and subtraction.

Final Considerations

Fundamental and simultaneously promising are the advances in studies that seek to better understand the cognitive processes potentially important for the development of number sense and its relationship with other numerical processing skills. Such advances can provide subsidies for the development of consistent assessments capable of identifying students at risk of developing difficulties in that area and interventions that focus on the various competencies. These specific and general domains are deficient. Interventions must be based on scientific evidence, theoretical models, and empirical studies that analyze intervention effects. Similarly, intervention models that enable teachers to work with students in the classroom have an important function, as they transcend the walls of academic research and align practice with the school context.

References

American Psychiatric Association – APA. (2014). DSM-5: Manual diagnóstico e estatístico de transtornos mentais (5a Ed.) (Nascimento, M.I, trad.). Artmed.

Aragón- Mendizábal, E., Aguilar-Villagrán, M., Navarro-Guzmán, J. I., & Howell, R. (2017). Improving number sense in kindergarten children with low achievement in mathematics. *Anales de Psicología, 33*(2), 311–318. https://doi.org/10.6018/analesps.33.2.239391

Assis, E. F. (2018). Intervenção em princípios de contagem: quatro estudos com alunos do 1° ano do Ensino Fundamental dissertação. (Tese de Doutorado, Universidade Federal do Rio Grande do Sul).

Baker, S., Gersten, R., & Lee, D. (2002). A synthesis of empirical research on teaching mathematics to low-achieving students. *The Elementary School Journal, 103*, 51–73. https://doi.org/10.1086/499715

Bryant, D. P., Bryant, B. R., Vaughn, G. R. S., Pfannenstiel, K., Porterfield, J., & Gersten, R. (2011). Early numeracy intervention program for first-grade students with mathematics difficulties. *Exceptional Children, 78*(1), 7–23.

Bull, R., & Johnston, R. S. (1997). Children's arithmetical difficulties: Contributions from processing speed, item identification and short-term memory. *Journal of Experimental Child Psychology, 65*, 1–24.

Bull, R., & Lee, K. (2014). Executive functioning and mathematics achievement. *Child Development Perspective, 8*, 36–41. https://doi.org/10.1006/jecp.1996.2358

Chen, X., Ye, M., Chang, L., Chen, W., & Zhou, R. (2018). Effect of working memory updating training on retrieving symptoms of children with learning disabilities. *Journal of Learning Disabilities, 51*(5), 507–519. https://doi.org/10.1006/jecp.1996.2358

Corso, L. V. (2018). Memória de trabalho, senso numérico e desempenho em aritmética. *Revista de Psicologia: Teoria e Prática, 20*(1), 141–154. https://doi.org/10.5935/1980-6906

Corso, L. V., & Assis, E. F. (2017). Reflexões acerca da aprendizagem inicial da matemática: contribuições de aspectos externos ao aluno. In L. Piccoli, L. V. Corso, S. S. Andrade, & R. Sperrhake (Eds.), *Pacto Nacional pela Alfabetização na Idade Certa PNAIC UFRGS: práticas de alfabetização, aprendizagem da matemática e políticas públicas* (1st ed., pp. 114–138). Oikos.

Corso, L., & Dorneles, B. (2010). Senso numérico e dificuldades de aprendizagem na matemática. *Revista Psicopedagogia, 27*(83), 298–309.

Corso, L. V., & Dorneles, B. V. (2012). Qual o papel que a memória de trabalho exerce na aprendizagem da Matemática. *Bolema. Boletim de Educação Matemática, 26*(42b), 627–647. https://doi.org/10.1590/S0103

Corso, L. V., & Dorneles, B. V. (2013). Avaliação da Matemática: competências numéricas e competências de base. In R. M. J. Scicchitano & M. I. S. Castanho (Eds.), *Avaliação Psicopedagógica: Recursos para a prática* (pp. 161–193). WAK editora.

Corso, L. V., & Dorneles, B. V. (2014). A velocidade de processamento e as dificuldades de aprendizagem na aritmética. *Estudos e Pesquisas em Psicologia, 14*, 949–966. https://doi.org/10.12957/epp.2014.13893

Corso, L. V., & Dorneles, B. V. (2015). Perfil cognitivo dos alunos com dificuldades de aprendizagem na leitura e matemática. *Psicologia: Teoria e Prática, 17*, 185–198. https://doi.org/10.15348/1980-6906

Cragg, L., Cragg, L., Keeble, S., Richardson, S., Roome, H., & Gilmore, C. (2017). Direct and indirect influences of executive functions on mathematics achievement. *Cognition, 162*, 12–26. https://doi.org/10.1016/j.cognition.2017.01.014

De Smedt, B., & Gilmore, C. (2011). Defective number module or impaired access? Numerical magnitude processing in first graders with mathematical difficulties. *Journal of experimental child psychology, 108*(2), 278–292. https://doi.org/10.1016/j.jecp.2010.09.003

Dehaene, S. (2001). Précis of the number sense. *Mind & Language, 16*, 16–36.

Dehaene, S., & Cohen, L. (1995). Towards an anatomical and functional model of number processing. *Mathematical Cognition, 1*, 83–120.

Dorneles, B. V., & Haase, V. G. (2017). Aprendizagem numérica em diálogo: neurociências e educação. In R. Lent, A. Buchweitz, & M. B. Mota (Eds.), *Ciência para Educação: uma ponte entre dois mundos* (pp. 133–160). Editora Atheneu.

Dowker, A. (2005). Early identification and interventions for students with mathematics difficulties. *Journal of Learning Disabilities, 38*(4), 324–332. https://doi.org/10.1177/00222194050380040801

Dyson, N., Jordan, N., & Glutting, J. (2011). A number sense intervention for low- income kindergartners at risk for mathematics difficulties. *Journal of Learning Disabilities, 42*(2), 166–181. https://doi.org/10.1177/0022219411410233

Friso-van den Bos, I., Van Der Ven, S., Kroesbergen, E., & Van Luit, J. (2013). Working memory and mathematics in primary school children: A meta-analysis. *Educational Research Review, 10*, 29–44. https://doi.org/10.1016/j.edurev.2013.05.003

Fuchs, L. S., Fuchs, D., Powell, S. R., Seethaler, P. M., Cirino, P. T., & Fletcher, J. M. (2008). Intensive intervention for students with mathematics disabilities: Seven principles of effective practice. *Learning Disabilities Quarterly, 38*(2), 79–92.

Fuchs, L. S., Geary, D. C., Schatscheneide, C., Hamlett, C. L., Deselms, J., Seethaler, P. M., Wilson, J., Craddock, C. F., Bryant, J. D., Luther, K., & Changas, P. (2013). Effects of first-grade number knowledge tutoring with contrasting forms of practice. *Journal of Educational Psychology, 105*(1), 58–77. https://doi.org/10.1037/a0030127

Fuchs, L. S., Powell, S. R., Seethaler, P. M., Cirino, P. T., Fletcher, J. M., Fuchs, D., & Hamlett, C. L. (2010). The effects of strategic counting instruction, with and without deliberate practice, on number combination skill among students with mathematics difficulties. *Learning Individual Differences, 20*(2), 89–100. https://doi.org/10.1016/j.lindif.2009.09.003

Geary, D. (2011). Consequences, characteristics, and causes of mathematical learning disabilities and persistent low achievement in mathematics. *Journal of Developmental & Behavioral Pediatrics, 32*(3), 250–263. https://doi.org/10.1097/DBP.0b013e318209edef

Gersten, R., & Chard, D. (1999). Number sense: rethinking arithmetic instruction for students with mathematical disabilities. *Journal of Special Education., 33*(1), 18–28. https://doi.org/10.1177/002246699903300102

Gersten, R., Jordan, N., & Flojo, J. (2005). Early identification and interventions for students with mathematics difficulties. *Journal of Learning Disabilities, 38*(4), 293–304. https://doi.org/10.1177/00222194050380040301

Greeno, J. G. (1991). Number sense as situated knowing in a conceptual domain. *Journal of Research in Mathematics Education, 23*(3), 170–218.

Haase, V. G., Costa, A. J., & Santos, F. H. (2015). Discalculia do desenvolvimento. In F. H. Santos, V. M. Andrade, & O. F. A. Bueno (Eds.), *Neuropsicologia Hoje* (pp. 160–168). Artmed.

Haase, V. G., Costa, A. J., Antunes, A. M., & Alves, I. S. (2012). Heterogeneidade cognitiva nas dificuldades de aprendizagem da matemática: Uma revisão bibliográfica. *PsicologiaemPesquisa, 6*(2), 139–150. https://doi.org/10.5327/Z1982-12472012000200007

Hecht, S., Torgesen, J., Wagner, R., & Rashotte, C. A. (2001). The Relations between phonological processing abilities and emerging individual differences in mathematical computation skills: A longitudinal study from second to fifth grades. *Journal of Experimental Child Psychology, 79*, 192–227. https://doi.org/10.1006/jecp.2000.2586

Jordan, N. C., Glutting, J., Ramineni, C., & Watkins, M. W. (2010). Validating a number sense screening tool for use in kindergarten and first grade: Prediction of mathematics proficiency in third grade. *School Psychology Review, 39*, 181–185.

Käser, T., Baschera, G. M., Kohn, J., Kucian, K., Richtmann, V., Grond, U., Gross, M., & von Aster, M. (2013). Design and evaluation of the computer-based training program Calcularis for enhancing numerical cognition. *Frontiers in Psychology, 4*, 1–13. https://doi.org/10.3389/fpsyg.2013.00489

Kroesbergen, E., Van Luit, J., Van Lieshout, E., Van Loosbroek, E., & Van De Rijt, B. (2009). Individual differences in early numeracy: The role of executive functions and subitizing. *Journal of Psychoeducational Assessment, 27*, 226–236. https://doi.org/10.1177/0734282908330586

Kucian, K., Grond, U., Rotzer, S., Henzi, B., Schönmann, C., Plangger, F., Gälli, M., Martin, E., & von Aster, M. (2011). Mental number line training in children with developmental dyscalculia. *NeuroImage, 57*, 782–795. https://doi.org/10.1016/j.neuroimage.2011.01.070

Kuhn, J., & Holling, H. (2014). Number sense or working memory? The effect of two computer-based trainings on mathematical skills in elementary school. *Advances in Cognitive Psychology, 10*(2), 59–67. https://doi.org/10.5709/acp-0157-2

Lee, K., Ng, S. F., Pe, M. L., Ang, S. Y., Hasshim, M. N., & Bull, R. (2012). The cognitive underpinnings of emerging mathematical skills: Executive functioning, patterns, numeracy, and arithmetic. *British Journal of Educational Psychology, 82*(1), 82–99. https://doi.org/10.1111/j.2044-8279.2010.02016.x

Melby-Lervag, M., & Hulme, C. (2013). Is working memory training effective? *A meta-analytic review. Developmental Psychology, 49*(2), 270–291. https://doi.org/10.1037/a0028228

Nelson, G., & Powell, S. (2017). A systematic review of longitudinal studies of mathematics difficulty. *Journal of Learning Disabilities, 51*(6), 523–539. https://doi.org/10.1177/0022219417714773

Nunes, T. (2009). Teacher notes. Department of Education – University of Oxford.

Nunes, T., & Moreno, C. (2002). An intervention program for promoting deaf pupils' achievement in mathematics. *Journal of Deaf Studies and Deaf Education, 7*(2), 120–133.

Nunes, T., Campos, T., Magina, S., & Bryant, P. (2005). *Educação Matemática: números e operações numéricas*. Cortez.

Nunes, T., Barros, R., Evans, D., & Burman, D. (2014). Improving deaf children's working memory through training. *International Journal of Speech & Language Pathology and Audiology, 2*(2), 51–66.

OECD. (2016). PISA 2015 Assessment and Analytical Framework: Science, Reading, Mathematic and Financial Literacy. PISA 2015 Mathematics Framework. PISA, OECD Publishing.

Okamoto, Y., & Case, R. (1996). Exploring the microstructure of children's central conceptual structures in the domain of number. *Monographs of the Society for Research in Child Development, 61*, 27–59.

Passolunghi, M., & Lanfranchi, S. (2012). Domain specific and domain general precursors of mathematical achievement: A longitudinal study from kindergarten to first grade. *British Journal of Educational Psychology, 82*, 42–63. https://doi.org/10.1111/j.2044-8279.2011.02039.x

Piccolo, L. R., Giacomoni, C. H., Julio-Costa, A., Oliveira, S., Zbornik, J., Haase, V. G., & Salles, J. F. (2017). Reading anxiety in L1: reviewing the concept. *Early Childhood Education Journal, 45*(4), 537–543.

Praet, M., & Desoete, A. (2014). Enhancing young children's arithmetic skills through non-intensive, computerized kindergarten interventions: A randomized controlled study. *Teaching and Teacher Education, 39*, 56–65. https://doi.org/10.1016/j.tate.2013.12.003

Santos, F. H. (2017). *Guia do Tutor Calcularis*. Pearson.

Silva, J. B. L., Moura, R. J., Wood, G., & Haase, V. G. (2015a). Processamento fonológico e desempenho em aritmética: uma revisão da relevância para as dificuldades de aprendizagem. *Temas em Psicologia, 23*(1), 157–173. https://doi.org/10.9788/TP2015.1-11

Silva, P. A., Ribeiro, F. S., & Santos, F. H. (2015b). Cognição numérica em crianças com transtorno específico de aprendizagem. *Temas em Psicologia, 23*(1), 197–210. https://doi.org/10.9788/TP2015.1-13

Sperafico, Y. L. (2016). Combined Intervention in Working Memory and Arithmetic Reasoning in Students With ADHD. (Tese de doutorado, Universidade Federal do Rio Grande do Sul).

Stock, P., Desoete, A., & Roeyers, H. (2009). Mastery of the counting principles in toddlers: A crucial step in the development of budding arithmetic abilities? *Learning and Individual Differences, 19*, 419–422. https://doi.org/10.1016/j.lindif.2009.03.002

Tolar, T. D., Fuchs, L., Fletcher, J. M., Fuchs, D., & Hamlett, C. L. (2016). Cognitive profiles of mathematical problem solving learning disability for different definitions of disability. *Journal of Learning Disabilities, 49*(3), 240–256. https://doi.org/10.1177/0022219414538520

Toll, S. W., Van der Ven, S. H., Kroesbergen, E. H., & Van Luit, J. E. (2011). Executive functions as predictors of math learning disabilities. *Journal of Learning Disabilities, 44*, 521–532. https://doi.org/10.1177/0022219410387302

Toll, S. W. (2013). A journey towards mathematics: Effects of remedial education on early numeracy. *Utrecht: Utrecht University Repository, 26*(4), 137–166.

Wilson, A. J., Dehaene, S., Pinel, P., Revkin, S. K., Cohen, L., & Cohen, D. (2006). Principles underlying the design of "the number race", an adaptive computer game for remediation of dyscalculia. *Behavioral and Brain Functions, 2*(1), 1–14. https://doi.org/10.1186/1744-9081-2-19

Chapter 13
Intervention in Reading Comprehension Skills

Helena Vellinho Corso, Luciana Vellinho Corso, and Jerusa Fumagalli de Salles

Reading skills can be studied at the levels of word recognition, fluency in decoding and textual reading, and reading comprehension. This chapter will focus on the more complex processes of reading (comprehension), which depend on all the others. On the other hand, reading comprehension is, in itself, a condition for the development of academic, professional, and even personal life of individuals. The Organization for Economic Cooperation and Development (OECD) broadly defines this skill as the ability to understand, use, reflect on, and engage with written texts to achieve goals, develop knowledge and potential, and participate in society (OECD, 1999).

Even with formal instruction, many children and adolescents do not achieve functional levels of comprehension, which negatively impacts their school performance and occupational future. This reality is forged from an early age, as lagging performances in reading (academic area of Portuguese) appear already at the beginning of the school journey (OECD, 2016).

Increasingly, effective intervention is being pointed out as a key component of the development of the ability to understand from reading (Connor, 2016). So much so that the latest edition of the DSM-5 diagnostic manual (APA, 2014) incorporates the response to instruction model as a diagnostic criterion for learning disorders. The symptom that specifies this disorder in the domain of reading comprehension is described in the manual as difficulties in understanding the meaning of what is read (that is, one can read a text correctly but not understand the sequence, relationships, inferences, or deeper meanings of what is read). The complexity of reading comprehension skills and the serious impairments caused by difficulties in this domain indicate the importance of preventive and remedial interventions, the topic of this chapter.

H. V. Corso (✉) · L. V. Corso · J. F. de Salles
Universidade Federal do Rio Grande do Sul, Porto Alegre, Brazil
e-mail: hvcorso@gmail.com; l.corso@terra.com.br; jerusafsalles@gmail.com

C. O. Cardoso, N. M. Dias (eds.), *Neuropsychological Interventions for Children - Volume 1*, https://doi.org/10.1007/978-3-031-53586-4_13

Reading Comprehension

Reading comprehension depends on the execution and integration of many cognitive and linguistic processes. To understand a sentence, the reader needs to visually process individual words, identify and access their phonological, orthographic, and semantic representations, and connect these representations to form an understanding of the meaning underlying the sentence. Similarly, to understand the text as a whole, the reader needs to process and connect individual idea units, resulting in the construction of a coherent mental representation of the text in the reader's memory (Kendeou et al., 2014). Kintsch (1998) highlights the interactive nature of the comprehension process, as the elements that make up this mental representation—in his theory called the situation model—come both from the text, via word perception, and from the reader himself, in the form of memories, knowledge, beliefs, or goals. In his construction-integration model, bottom-up processes (i.e., from the text to the reader) are complemented by top-down processes (i.e., from the reader to the text), which select, abstract, and organize a coherent global structure or a network of meanings. The construction, from initially decontextualized elements, is followed by the process that restricts information, according to prior knowledge, integrating it. In this sense, the author considers that comprehension, understood as this interactive text-reader process, functions as a paradigm for cognition as a whole, involving the most general cognitive processes, such as working memory, problem-solving, and learning.

Making inferences is a fundamental component to arrive at a coherent mental representation of the text, and at least two important types of inferences can be identified: those that join the distinct elements of the text (for example, a pronoun and its referent; example: *He was happy when he saw him arrive*) to construct cohesion and internal coherence, through passive inferential processes (occur automatically); and those that connect textual information and the reader's prior knowledge through strategic inferential processes (example: *He was near the area, so he kicked the ball hard to score a goal*; in the example, the reader uses his prior knowledge to infer that the subject would be playing soccer, but the information is not explicitly stated in the text), which demand attention and working memory (WM) resources from the reader. The study by Richard et al. (2014) showed that executive functions (EF) are specifically recruited for elaborative (strategic) inferences, as it found a significant association between WM tasks, monitoring, and cognitive flexibility and this type of inference. This association was not evidenced with bridge inferences (automatic) or weakly (and only with WM tasks).

Different authors have been emphasizing the role of school instruction in the development of the ability to understand a text since reading comprehension strategies need to be taught (Colomer & Camps, 2002; Solé, 1998), greatly impacting the reader's performance. Indeed, in Connor's (2016) comprehension development model, which already gathers consistent evidence, instruction plays a central role, interacting with the factors already mentioned. It is a network model that describes reading comprehension as a complex activity that requires the reader to coordinate

1. Specific text processes (fluency in decoding and encoding and the structure of the text)
2. Socio-emotional and cognitive processes (these form a single system, which includes motivation and the regulatory processes involved in learning: EF and metacognition)
3. Linguistic processes (which include the lexical system—knowledge of words; the semantic system—including academic knowledge; syntax—grammar; morphology; and oral language comprehension)
4. Instruction

The first three processes develop over time, interact with each other, have a reciprocal boosting effect, and are affected by instruction (at school and home). This is also affected by the first processes, as children develop physically, linguistically, socially, cognitively, and emotionally throughout early and middle childhood, which also influences learning and the effectiveness of instruction. These processes are malleable but respond to different influences to varying degrees and may be more malleable earlier in childhood than later.

As for comprehension difficulty, its main manifestations are failures to recall the main ideas of the read text, failures to answer literal or inferential questions about it, and difficulty in finishing reading the text. Such failures may be due to deficits in low-level processes (such as decoding, reading fluency, and vocabulary knowledge, which translate the written code into meaningful language units), high-level processes (such as making strategic inferences through executive functioning, which allows organizing and reflecting on information within the limits of working memory capacity), or both. Identifying the causes helps define the appropriate instructional material and the type of intervention needed to remedy the source of difficulty (Kendeou et al., 2014).

While it is true that failures in word recognition and fluency negatively affect comprehension, it is also a fact that difficulty in understanding can occur in the absence of problems in these more basic processes. The specific difficulty in reading comprehension corresponds precisely to the difficulty of accessing the meaning of the text, with fluent decoding processes preserved. Therefore, in research on comprehension difficulties, it is necessary to formally evaluate the word recognition ability, which should be in a medium performance range (Fletcher et al., 2009). As for the prevalence of this specific difficulty, most studies, mainly American and European, produce estimates between 5% and 10%, depending on the exclusion criteria and cut-off points used (Fletcher et al., 2009). A Brazilian study (Corso et al., 2013b) produced an even higher estimate: the clear dissociation between the ability to recognize the word (preserved) and the ability to understand the read text (impaired) was verified in 17% of the sample ($n = 110$; 9–12 years; public and private schools).

According to the DSM-5 (APA, 2014), the difficulty in understanding the meaning of what is read can be diagnosed as a learning disorder with a specific symptom in this subdomain of reading, provided that the impairment in this academic skill persists for at least 6 months despite interventions aimed at the difficulties. Other diagnostic criteria are as follows: the affected skills are below what is expected for chronological age and interfere with academic performance; the difficulties begin during school years. Other disorders or deficiencies, psychosocial adversity, lack of proficiency in the language of academic instruction, or inadequate educational instruction cannot better explain the difficulties).

The different components of the construct reading comprehension and its latent nature determine difficulties and care in assessing the skill (Corso et al., 2017). On the other hand, reliable and comprehensive assessment is an indispensable condition for the intervention that is intended to be effective in the face of reading comprehension difficulties.

Intervention of Reading Comprehension Skills in Childhood

Some authors have drawn attention to the importance of unifying research on learning disorders and the development of the skills in question. This is what happens, for example, in the case of reading research at the word recognition level, where the same theory that explains how the child develops the ability to recognize the word explains why some fail, which occurs in dyslexia (Fletcher et al., 2009). As we have seen, we also already have some important advances in the scientific understanding of reading at the level of comprehension. It is expected that these comprehensive models of reading comprehension skills will increasingly serve as a basis to guide not only rehabilitation in the face of difficulties but also to underpin educational practices that can prevent them by stimulating the development of the skill.

While at the word recognition level the cognitive/neuropsychological components with the most consistent scientific evidence are the phonological processing skills of language (Corso & Dorneles, 2015), numerous studies have been pointing to EF as a key component for reading comprehension (Salles & Paula, 2016). In a neuropsychological assessment battery covering eight functions, it was the tasks of WM (Visuospatial working memory, with strong participation of the executive component: the participant had to maintain the sequence of cubes pointed out by the examiner, simultaneously to the inversion of the presented series) and EF (orthographic and semantic verbal fluency) that differentiated the groups of good and poor comprehenders (Corso et al., 2013c). A study (Corso et al., 2016) using structural equation modeling to test the different relationships between socioeconomic level (SES), intelligence and EF (independent variables) on reading comprehension showed that not only do EF have a direct effect on reading comprehension, but they mediate the relationship between SES and comprehension, while intelligence did not show a significant effect on reading comprehension. In this study, SES explained 31% of the variance in EF, which, in turn, was responsible for explaining 52% of the variance in reading comprehension.

In the two subsections below, we will address the intervention in reading comprehension in remedial and preventive contexts. It is essential that clinical and school practices are based on scientific knowledge, overcoming intuitive paths towards systematic interventions with proven efficacy. In this sense, we will seek to present research evidence for the suggestions and strategies presented. As we will see, the EF and metacognitive skills—concepts that have a close relationship (Corso et al., 2013a), are contemplated in several of these suggestions and strategies.

Intervention in Reading Comprehension Skills in a Remedial Context

Specific Learning Disorder is defined as a neurodevelopmental disorder of biological origin, which is the basis for abnormalities at the cognitive level, which in turn are associated with the behavioral signs of the disorder. The biological origin includes an interaction of genetic, epigenetic and environmental factors, which affect the brain's ability to perceive or process verbal or non-verbal information efficiently and accurately (APA, 2014). The idea of improving a skill that rests on certain neurobiological bases relies on a certain conception about the constitution and development of such bases (Corso & Salles, 2017). Within an interactionist development model, the neurobiological bases of learning are not seen as innate or emerging according to a maturational timetable—a view that would imply a direction of causality in one direction, from the brain to behavior. On the contrary, the relationship between the brain and behavior is seen as bidirectional (Pennington, 2009). Confirming the interactionist models of development and learning, intensive and explicit interventions with children with significant reading difficulties, including dyslexia and comprehension difficulties, have proven to be quite effective (Torgesen, 2005).

The EF, central to the process of text comprehension, are malleable and, therefore, susceptible to development under stimulation and training (for more information on EF, see Chap. 9 of this work). A review article (Karbach & Unger, 2014) reveals the increase in scientific studies on EF training since these cognitive functions are pointed out as predictors of various achievements throughout life, such as academic performance, socioeconomic level and physical health. The focus on training in children and adolescents is justified because behavioral and neural plasticity is particularly high in childhood, as the frontal lobes, responsible for EF, are highly sensitive to environmental stimuli. Most of the studies analyzed showed significant improvements in performance on the trained tasks, which opens the doors for possible interventions, both educational and therapeutic.

Several programs have already been evaluated regarding EF training aimed at the development and/or rehabilitation of reading comprehension. Garcia-Madruga et al. (2013) empirically tested a training program in executive processes of WM aimed at increasing reading comprehension. Two experiments were conducted with 3rd-grade elementary school children. In the first, the experimental group showed greater gains in both comprehension and intelligence measures. In the second, the effect of training on two groups—high and low performance in comprehension in the pre-test—was compared. The results showed significant improvements in comprehension, intelligence, and executive processes, with the low-performance group achieving greater gains than the high performance group. The study by Coelho and Correa (2010) evaluated the effect of training monitoring skills on comprehension ability using the methodology of the error detection paradigm: the adolescents (9th grade of Elementary School) in the experimental group were asked to systematically look for errors (lexical level) and inconsistencies (level of integration of ideas) in the texts read, correct such errors and reread the text so that the two basic processes of monitoring—detection and regulation—were contemplated. After the intervention, the experimental group was significantly better than the control group in reading and monitoring tasks. In addition, it was observed that, during the intervention process, the students gradually became more interested and attentive to their reading, promoting not only comprehension but also motivation for reading.

Research like this indicates important directions that clinical practice should consider. In the clinical context, however, the enhancement of EF may require a specific approach, as it also considers the subjectivity and history of the individual, which need to be taken into account in defining therapeutic paths available or to be created. Such paths can encompass all domains of EF at once, in service of expressive and creative tasks, which ensure the necessary motivation by involving the patient's subjectivity. Reports of clinical case studies show the improvement of patients with difficulties in reading comprehension through a psychopedagogical therapeutic technique that develops EF—the model building (Corso, 2017; Corso et al., 2018). The construction of a model starts from an idea of the patient, who defines the object, place, and scene they would like to represent (more or less completely) through scaled-down construction. After the idea is conceived, planning begins. It is supervised by the therapist and written on a card developed especially for this, including elements, materials, spatial location, etc. Usually, the model building is done on a styrofoam base, and all the other elements are assembled/modeled (according to the material used) in three dimensions. Gradually, over several sessions, the different elements conceived by the patient are being built, with more or less help from the therapist, depending on the patient's need (Corso et al., 2018).

Intervention in Reading Comprehension Skills in a Preventive Context

The school is, without a doubt, a fundamental space for the prevention of comprehension difficulties through pedagogical approaches that promote the development of the skill. The public school, in particular, which receives students from a low socioeconomic level, has an important role in this regard, as this factor can translate into a risk factor for reading performance.

Morais et al. (2013) cite different studies showing that before being taught to read, children's readiness for learning to read is already heavily influenced by the sociocultural environment in which they grew up and find themselves. Children who begin learning to read in schools in a favored sociocultural environment are, on average, already much more advanced than those who attend schools in a disadvantaged environment. In the following years, these differences persist, so much so that, compared to children from favored environment schools, most children from disadvantaged environments, even with good relative results in their school, appear to be poor readers. Citing results from longitudinal studies, the authors conclude that a child from a socially disadvantaged environment is seven to eight times more likely to become a poor reader than a child from a favored environment.

A study (Corso et al., 2013b) that evaluated students' reading from 4th grade to 6th grade showed a significant effect of the variable 'type of school' (public *versus* private). Both in the task of reading isolated words and in the instrument used to assess reading comprehension, the performance of public school students in all three grades was significantly lower than that of private school children.

Thus, reading comprehension intervention programs aimed at stimulating the learning of this skill become especially important, or even crucial, for students from disadvantaged classes to reduce the gap produced by an unfavorable environment. The study by Fonseca et al. (2014) evaluated the impact, among children from schools of different socioeconomic levels, of a program developed from four components of reading comprehension: vocabulary, construction of inferences, monitoring, and understanding of textual structure. The program consists of 16 units of increasing complexity developed from an expository or narrative text. The activities on the texts are organized in three moments: "Before reading" (vocabulary is worked on, activation of prior knowledge and making predictions); "Active reading" (students are taught to monitor their own understanding, recognizing the new information from the text and detecting when they fail to understand); and "After reading" (students learn to answer questions, to use graphic organizers, to identify main and secondary ideas, and to summarize in topics). The different strategies are mediated by the teacher, who teaches the key concepts: he demonstrates how and when to apply the strategies and assists the children until they can appropriate them and use them autonomously. Following a pre and post-test design in two groups (intervention and control) within each of two distinct schools (low socioeconomic level and medium socioeconomic level), significant improvements were observed in both groups in relation to their controls in vocabulary, comprehension of texts, construction of inferences and monitoring, proving the importance of explicit teaching of strategies and the need for systematic work on the program's axes.

In an exhaustive review, Fletcher et al. (2009) verified two types of reading comprehension intervention programs—those focused on specific skills, considered components of reading comprehension (such as vocabulary or morphological awareness), and those focused on cognitive strategies, concluding that the most effective methods are those centered on strategy instructions. As the authors point out, from the examination of different studies, a central aspect of both types of intervention is the idea that instruction should be explicit, contradicting the common sense notion, also present among teachers, that reading a lot can improve comprehension by itself. Students need to be taught to analyze and think about what they have read to understand the text's deep meaning. Moreover, the examination of comprehension strategies shows that they involve, exactly, executive functions, since they involve the establishment of conscious objectives, planning and self-monitoring (Corso & Salles, 2017).

It is desirable that public policies incorporate the concern of reducing the disadvantage of low socioeconomic level children in the development of text comprehension skills, as much as it is desirable that implemented programs have proven efficacy. In the United States, there has been a concern that educators use pedagogical approaches whose efficiency has scientific proof. The American Department of Education created a fund—*What Works Clearinghouse*[1]—to conduct increasingly rigorous studies that evaluate what really works in various areas and stages of education. For example, a study (James-Burdumy et al., 2010) evaluated the impact of four curriculum programs (Project CRISS, *Read About, Read for Real, Reading for Knowledge*) designed to enhance reading comprehension skills. The randomized controlled study included more than 5500 5th-grade students attending 89 schools in 10 high-poverty school districts. Within each of the ten districts, schools were randomly assigned to one of the four intervention groups that received one of the supplementary curricula or to the control group that received no supplementary curriculum. The four curricula under review were systematized by different authors/universities and, with minor variations (such as the type of texts used; the curriculum support material—textbooks or computer program), encompass the teaching of strategies (such as summarizing and finding the main idea) and focus on some specific skills (such as vocabulary and fluency).

Students who used the supplementary curricula did not score higher in reading comprehension than students who did not use these curricula. Interestingly, the study found statistically significant associations between the low scores of students who received the supplementary curriculum, on the one hand, and certain characteristics of the students, teachers, or schools, on the other. Thus, in the intervention groups, students who at baseline showed reading fluency levels below the expected average, students with baseline comprehension levels in the bottom third of the sample, and students eligible for free meal programs showed lower performances. There was also a correlation between the low performance of students who received the supplementary curriculum and the school's score on the school professional culture scale (which reflects teachers' perceptions about the culture in the school, including relationships with colleagues, access to professional development, experiences with changes being implemented in their school, and leadership support in their schools). These results seem to confirm Connor's (2016) model, in which the reciprocal effect between cognitive, linguistic, and developmental aspects of children and instruction is seen so that if the intervention impacts those developments, the effect it achieves is also modulated by them. It is concluded that ensuring the full development of language in general, and initial reading in particular, is fundamental for these students to have cognitive and linguistic resources to take advantage of

[1] *What Works Clearinghouse:* https://ies.ed.gov/ncee/wwc/

their own reading comprehension intervention programs. Similarly, the teacher—a key piece of the instructional process—also influences the effect of the curriculum programs through their training, values, and professional opportunities offered by their school.

Reading Comprehension Intervention—Main Topics

- There is sufficient evidence that intensive and explicit interventions with children with significant reading difficulties, including comprehension difficulties, have proven to be quite effective.
- Reading comprehension skill is complex and multicomponent, so interventions in comprehensive reading can focus on different components. Different reading comprehension intervention programs aimed at stimulating the learning of this skill have been tested with different types of schools/students/grades in different countries. Generally, instruction in one or more specific components of comprehension (for example, vocabulary and morphological awareness) and those focused on teaching reading strategies have proven to be efficient.
- The teaching of strategies involves those to be used before reading (such as activation of prior knowledge, for example), during reading (such as monitoring to identify passages not understood), and after reading (such as identification of main ideas).
- A central aspect of any intervention—school or clinical—is the idea that instruction should be explicit.
- According to consistent research findings, EF and metacognition (that is, regulatory processes) are key elements of the ability to understand texts, which suggests that focusing on these functions at the level of neuropsychological rehabilitation of the skill can favor the development of reading comprehension.
- Various EF training programs aimed at developing and/or re(ha)bilitation of reading comprehension have already been evaluated, proving effective.
- In the clinic (psychopedagogical or neuropsychological), it is possible to develop both the strategies usable in the classroom and more expressive and creative tasks, which involve more directly the patient's subjectivity in developing the EF, such as model building.
- Specific and direct work with reading processes is fundamental for the success of the intervention, whether or not it is associated with the intervention in skills related to reading.

Final Considerations

In this chapter we addressed the intervention in reading comprehension in school (preventive) and clinical (remedial) contexts. As we sought to demonstrate, it is essential that all practice aimed at the enhancement of the reading comprehension skill is based on scientific knowledge, both of the models of processing and development of reading, as well as scientifically designed studies of intervention efficacy, constituting systematic interventions, with proven efficacy. Hence, studies conducted in the area of comprehension are important. Although there is still much to be done, the research results in this field are already quite promising. The dissemination of this knowledge and the circulation of this information is key so that all professionals (teachers, psychopedagogues, psychologists, speech therapists, etc.) whose practice involves this skill in their student/patient can overcome intuitive approaches, replacing them with effective interventions.

References

American Psychiatric Association – APA. (2014). Manual diagnóstico e estatístico de transtornos mentais. (5a ed., tradução: Maria Inês Corrêa Nascimento et al.). Artmed.

Coelho, C., & Correa, J. (2010). Desenvolvimento da Compreensão Leitora através do Monitoramento da Leitura. *Psicologia: Reflexão e Crítica, 23*(3), 575–581. https://doi.org/10.1590/S0102-79722010000300018

Colomer, T., & Camps, A. (2002). *Ensinar a ler, ensinar a compreender*. Artmed.

Connor, C. M. (2016). A lattice model of the development of reading comprehension. *Child Development Perspectives, 10*(4), 269–274. https://doi.org/10.1111/cdep.12200

Corso, H. V. (2017). Avaliação da dificuldade de compreensão leitora: um caso da clínica psicopedagógica. In H. V. Corso, L. Piccolo, C. Mina, & J. F. Salles (Eds.), *Avaliação da compreensão da leitura textual (COMTEXT): para crianças do 4° ao 6° ano do ensino fundamental* (pp. 83–100). Vetor.

Corso, L. V., & Dorneles, B. V. (2015). Perfil cognitivo dos alunos com dificuldades de aprendizagem na leitura e matemática. *Revista Psicologia: Teoria e Prática, 17*(2), 185–198. https://doi.org/10.15348/1980-6906/psicologia.v17n2p185-198

Corso, H. V., Cromley, J. G., Sperb, T., & Salles, J. F. (2016). Modeling the relationship among reading comprehension. Intelligence, socioeconomic status, and neuropsychological functions: The mediating role of executive functions. *Psychology & Neuroscience, 9*, 1–14. https://doi.org/10.1037/pne0000036

Corso, H. V., Jou, G. I., Cortez, T., & Forner, V. (2018). Treinamento do controle executivo no contexto da pesquisa e da clínica psicopedagógica. In N. T. Rotta, C. A. Bridi Filho, & F. R. Bridi (Eds.), *Plasticidade Cerebral e Aprendizagem – abordagem multidisciplinar* (pp. 81–100). Artmed.

Corso, H. V., Jou, G. I., Sperb, T. M., & Salles, J. F. (2013a). "Metacognição" e "Funções Executivas": relações entre o conceito psicológico e neuropsicológico na perspectiva da aprendizagem. *Psicologia: Teoria e Pesquisa, 29*(1), 21–29. https://doi.org/10.1590/S0102-37722013000100004

Corso, H. V., Sperb, T. M., & Salles, J. F. (2013b). Leitura de palavras e de texto em crianças: efeitos de série e tipo de escola, e dissociações de desempenhos. *Letras de Hoje, 48*(1), 81–90.

Corso, H. V., Sperb, T. M., & Salles, J. F. (2013c). Comparison between poor comprehenders and good readers in neuropsychological tasks. *Psicologia em Pesquisa, 7*(1), 37–49. https://doi.org/10.5327/Z1982-1247201300010005

Corso, H. V., Piccolo, L., Mina, C., & Salles, J. F. (2017). *Avaliação da compreensão da leitura textual (COMTEXT): para crianças do 4° ao 6° ano do ensino fundamental*. Vetor.

Corso, H. V., & Salles, J. F. (2017). Reabilitação neuropsicológica das dificuldades específicas em compreensão leitora. In D. R. Fontoura, L. Tisser, O. Bueno, S. Bolognani, & T. Frison (Eds.), *Teoria e prática na reabilitação neuropsicológica* (pp. 219–239). Vetor.

Fletcher, J. M., Lyons, G. R., Fuchs, L. S., & Barnes, M. A. (2009). *Transtornos de aprendizagem – da identificação à intervenção*. Artmed.

Fonseca, L., Pujals, M., Lasala, E., Lagomarsino, I., Migliardo, G., Aldrey, A., Buonsanti, L., & Barreyro, J. P. (2014). Desarrollo de habilidades de comprensión lectora em niños de escuelas de distintos sectores socioeconómicos. *Neuropsicologia Latinoamericana, 6*(1), 41–50. https://doi.org/10.5579/rnl.2014.0151

García-Madruga, J. A., Elosúa, M. R., Gil, L., Gómez-Veiga, I., Vila, J. O., Orjales, I., Contreras, A., Rodríguez, R., Melero, M. A., & Duque, G. (2013). Reading comprehension and working memory's executive processes: An intervention study in primary school students. *Reading Research Quarterly, 48*(2), 155–174. https://doi.org/10.1002/rrq.44

James-Burdumy, S., Mansfield, W., Deke, J., Carey, N., Lugo-Gil, J., Hershey, A., Douglas, A., Gersten, R., Newman-Gonchar, R., Dimino, J., & Faddis, B. (2010). *Effectiveness of selected supplemental reading comprehension interventions: Impacts on a first cohort of fifth-grade students. What Works Clearinghouse*. Nacional center for Education Evaluation and Regional Assistance, Institute of Education Sciences, U. S. Department of Education.

Karbach, J., & Unger, K. (2014). Executive control training from middle childhood to adolescence. *Frontiers in Psychology, 5*. https://doi.org/10.3389/fpsyg.2014.00390

Kendeou, P., Van Den Broek, P., Helder, A., & Karlsson, J. (2014). A cognitive view of reading comprehension: Implications for reading difficulties. *Learning Disabilities Research & Practice, 29*(1), 10–16. https://doi.org/10.1111/ldrp.12025

Kintsch, W. (1998). *Comprehension: A paradigm for cognition*. Cambridge University Press.

Morais, J., Leite, I., & Kolinsky, R. (2013). Entre a pré-leitura e a leitura hábil: condições e patamares da aprendizagem. In M. R. Maluf & C. Cardoso-Martins (Eds.), *Alfabetização no Século XXI: Como se Aprende a Ler e a Escrever* (pp. 17–48). Penso.

Organization for Economic Cooperation and Development – OECD. (1999). *Measuring student knowledge and skills: A new framework for assessment*. OECD.

OECD. (2016). *PISA 2015 assessment and analytical framework: Science, reading, mathematic and financial literacy* (PISA). OECD Publishing.

Pennington, B. F. (2009). *Diagnosing learning disorders: A neuropsychological framework* (Vol. 2). The Guilford Press.

Richard's, M., Juric, L. C., Introzzi, I., & Urquijo, S. (2014). Differential intervention of executive functions in elaborative and bridging inferences. *Avances en Psicología Latinoamericana, 32*(1), 5–20. https://doi.org/10.12804/apl32.1.2014.01

Salles, J. F., & Paula, F. V. (2016). Text reading comprehension and its relationship with executive functions. *Educar em Revista, 62*, 53–67. https://doi.org/10.1590/0104-4060.48332

Solé, I. (1998). *Estratégias de leitura*. Artmed.

Torgesen, J. K. (2005). Recent discoveries on remedial interventions for children with dyslexia. In M. Snowling & C. Hulme (Eds.), *The science of reading: A handbook* (pp. 209–226). Blackwell.

Index

C. O. Cardoso, N. M. Dias (eds.), *Neuropsychological Interventions for Children - Volume 1*, https://doi.org/10.1007/978-3-031-53586-4